"When I was a little girl of four years of age, I had my tonsils out. On my way to the hospital, my mother, a nurse, told me exactly what procedures would happen in the surgery room. When these did occur exactly as she said, my fear subsided because I knew what to expect. Although every cancer patient's experience is unique in many ways, because Sharon Callister has shared so intimately her own journey of breast cancer, this book offers a gift similar to that my mother gave me—knowing what to expect."

Ruth Thomas
Professor, University of Minnesota

* * *

"A courageous reflection of a spiritual journey through breast cancer recovery. Her exploration of Christian faith during this process is insightful and instructive for all caregivers, both clergy and laity. God has truly blessed us through Sharon's writing with a deeper level of helpfulness to empathize with illness. Thank you, Sharon!"

Rev. Dr. Gary A. Titusdahl
First Congregational Church, UCC
Cannon Falls, MN

* * *

"Adversity is no respecter of the barriers of culture, social standing or belief. When an adversary, so personal as breast cancer, lodges close to home, support is needed. Greater succor is needed when such a wound is compounded be a mindset of silence, be it from one's national culture, which may diminish the voice of a woman, or from the stigma of such an intimate battle.

"Sharon provides liberation by giving a voice to all those impacted by this disease. Sharon Callister speaks for, not just the patient, but also one's spouse and supporters. With astonishing vividness, one is brought into the private world of the author. These devotionals will usher one through a journey that brings healing in its wings. I highly recommend this book to anyone who is facing the seemingly insurmountable challenge of cancer."

Edward Shawa, Senior Associate Pastor
Redeeming Love Church, AG,
St. Paul, MN

* * *

"This book honestly confronts the human emotion of a cancer diagnosis. Sharon aptly describes how breast cancer transformed her. Her faith bolstered her inner strength, increasing her courage to meet the challenges of a life-changing event. *On Wings of the Dawn* will offer strength and support to those facing cancer and their caregivers."

Leona Stevens, RN, BA, Breast Center Nurse Clinician,
providing oncology care since 1985.

On Wings of the Dawn

A devotional book for women experiencing breast cancer and their supporters

Sharon Callister

Hold tight to your mustard seed faith. God *is* faithful! Sharon Callister

Beaver's Pond Press, Inc.
Edina, Minnesota

Unless otherwise noted, Scripture quotations are from the New American Standard Bible, copyright © 1960, 1962, 1963,1968, 1971, 1972, 1973, 1975, 1977 The Lockman Foundation. Used by permission.

Scripture marked LB are taken from the Living Bible.

Scripture marked KJV are taken from the King James Version.

Scripture marked NIV are taken from the Holy Bible, New International version.

Scripture marked NSRV are taken from the New Revised Standard Version.

Scripture marked RSV are taken from the Revised Standard Version.

ISBN 1-59298-020-1

Library of Congress Catalog Number: 2003110546

Book design and typesetting: Mori Studio
Cover design: Mori Studio

Printed in the United States of America

First Printing: September 2003

06 05 04 03 6 5 4 3 2 1

Beaver's Pond Press, Inc.

7104 Ohms Lane, Suite 216
Edina, MN 55439
(952) 829-8818
www.BeaversPondPress.com

to order, visit *www.BookHouseFulfillment.com* or call 1-800-901-3480. Reseller discounts available.

This book is dedicated to my husband, Colin,
who, on our wedding day,
vowed to love and cherish me,
in sickness and in health—
and has kept his promise.

Table of Contents

Acknowledgements

It is with a grateful heart that I say "thank you" to these willing channels through whom God worked to help me bring readers *On Wings of the Dawn*:

My long-distance friend, Mary Marsh, who first introduced me to devotional books more than thirty years ago, and who has generously given me a devotional book almost every Christmas since. Because of my familiarity with the devotional style of writing and its ability to nurture spiritual growth, the writing of this book flowed naturally and passionately.

My longtime friend, Carol Compton, who always knew I would someday write a book, and who encouraged me to begin writing this book.

My husband, Colin, my mother, Edith Ailie, and my sisters, Carol Sangren and Janet Barberg—who became my most diligent cheering team while I wrote.

My family: Aaron, Krissy, Vince, Hudson, Matt, and Eric, who love me unconditionally, despite my idiosyncrasies.

My "prayer warriors"—especially Beth, Charlotte, Phyllis, Debbie, Gay, Julie, Holly, and Tammy—who prayed me through my seasons of breast cancer and writing.

My reviewers, Angela Callister, Ruth Thomas, and Gary Titusdahl, who spent hours reading and critiquing rough drafts.

The many women and men who expressed gratitude to me for the support they received from reading my "in progress" devotionals while undergoing cancer treatment. Their affirmation inspired me to continue writing.

My team of professionals who helped birth *On Wings of the Dawn:* My publisher, Milt Adams, who enthusiastically mentored me through the process; Hope LaVine, my editor, who guided me with a velvet glove through grammatical correctness and manuscript readability; my proofreader, Terri Hudoba, who made final corrections; and Jack Caravela and Jaana Bykonich at Mori Studio Inc., who caught my vision for the book's design and beautifully brought it to life.

And, finally but foremost, I give thanks, praise, and glory to God for this book, and for everything I am and hope to be.

Introduction

Sometimes the message of a book is revealed through the images that grace its cover. And so it is with this book.

A beautiful butterfly, lit on a daisy, basking in the dawn of a new day. Fix this image in your mind's eye as I introduce you to *On Wings of the Dawn.*

"He loves me, he loves me not. He loves me, He loves me not." One by one I'd pluck the petals off a daisy as I'd recite the familiar girlhood rhyme. The daisy—the cheery flower that had once whimsically disclosed the affections of boyfriends—became significant in a different way following my breast cancer diagnosis. The "he" was no longer my latest crush—but God. Did my diagnosis mean "God loves me?" or "God loves me not?" What would the final plucked petal reveal?

The message of Psalm 139 is that God knows each of us intimately, is with us at all times wherever we go, and lovingly leads us in His everlasting way. Over the years I'd enjoyed visualizing myself, as in verse 9, taking the "wings of the dawn" into each new day. But . . . sometimes the wings of a new day carry us to places we don't want to go. A first-hand experience with breast cancer is one of those places.

Verses 9 and 10 promise that even "If I dwell in the remotest part of the sea, even there Thy hand will lead me and Thy right hand will lay hold of me." Would God lead me through my "remotest part of the sea"—breast cancer treatments? Would I be held securely in His right hand throughout all the unknowns ahead?

A breast cancer diagnosis can feel like being trapped in a dark, ugly cocoon. When one observes a cocoon, it seems impossible that a beautiful butterfly could be forming within its confines.

Yet, in God's perfect time and way, such a butterfly does indeed appear. Is it possible that an amazing miracle can also take place within the "cocoon" of breast cancer? That in God's perfect time and way a transformed, beautiful woman can emerge?

These are among the images and questions that are addressed and answered with candor, intimacy, and honesty within the pages of *On Wings of the Dawn*. This is a book that has been conceived, developed, and born to meet the heart-and-soul cry of women who—like me—need and long for information, support, and hope beyond that offered by books that emphasize primarily the physical aspects of breast cancer.

When did I first realize that the resources pertaining to the physical impact of breast cancer were insufficient for the *whole* me—my mental, emotional, spiritual, and relational dimensions? It was on my diagnosis day as I drove home from the doctor's office—expressed succinctly in this brief excerpt from the devotional, "A Still Small Voice," that concludes the Diagnosis chapter:

"Jarred out of my whirlwind of thoughts by the realization that I was driving too fast, I looked at the speedometer: 75 miles per hour! I was thankful I hadn't been pulled over for speeding. What would I have told the law enforcement officer? "I'm driving under the influence of breast cancer"?

Yes, there is no doubt that breast cancer affects every aspect of a woman's life. By the time I had completed two surgeries and my first chemotherapy treatment, I was becoming desperate in my search for emotional and spiritual support. I drove to the nearest bookstore, walked up to the first employee I spotted, and asked, "Do you have a devotional book for women experiencing breast cancer?" "No" she replied, "but my mother died of breast cancer, and she needed that kind of book too. Why don't you write one?"

It is my belief that God knows the unanswered questions and unmet needs of women experiencing breast cancer and those who support them. By His grace and guidance, He has helped me write a book that not only gives voice to such questions and needs, but also provides an abundance of answers, support, and hope.

You may wonder why I have written this book in a devotional format. After years of reading daily, and other, devotional books, I have come to a realization—God's living word in Scripture, coupled with relationship-nurturing communication with Him through prayer, brings a ministry that transcends the sharing of human experience. With that in mind, I believe God will use these devotionals to reveal His nature and blessing to each reader on an individual, personal level.

That being said, this book is intended to be a vital source of support, not only for the Christian, but also for the non-Christian, for the skeptic, for those who perceive God as a She rather than a He, for those of any religion or no religion, and for people of all cultural and ethnic backgrounds.

Why is this book also intended for those who support women experiencing breast cancer? Because it provides a rare opportunity to vicariously share the breast cancer experience of the woman you love and care about:

- She could be your wife, mother, daughter, grandmother, granddaughter, sister, aunt, niece, cousin or in-law, fiancee, or significant other.
- She could be your friend, neighbor, co-worker, teacher, student, pastor, medical-care provider, or business associate.
- She could be your current or future patient, parishioner, client, employee, or customer.
- She could be you, in the event that you are someday diagnosed with breast cancer, wondering what it is really like to experience this disease.

The 2003 statistics reported by the American Cancer Society indicate that one out of eight American women will be diagnosed with breast cancer during her lifetime. Thankfully, great strides are being taken in the diagnosis and treatment of breast cancer—dramatically increasing the survival rate. Hopefully, a cure will be discovered soon. In the meantime, by gaining a glimpse into the world of breast cancer, you will be better prepared to face your own diagnosis, or to understand and support someone else who is so diagnosed.

On Wings of the Dawn is written in a manner that provides several reading options. The devotionals are organized to flow chronologically, so the book may be read from cover to cover. Some readers will choose to read the chapter or individual devotionals most pertinent to the phase of treatment being experienced currently or coming up next. Many, especially women whose course of treatment varies from mine, will prefer to use the subject index as a guide to the most relevant and helpful devotionals for any given day.

Finally, to satisfy your desire to know the "last page first," this is a victorious book. What does plucking the last daisy petal reveal? HE LOVES ME! The final petal triumphantly proclaims for all the world to hear that I know, that I know, that I know, that I know He loves me—like I never knew before, and may have never known had I not ridden the wings of the dawn to a breast cancer diagnosis.

Be assured, dear reader, that you are God's beloved child. Wherever the wings of the dawn take you, God will hold you securely in His hand and lead you through whatever the day brings. Your breast cancer experience doesn't have to be a wasted season in your life, but rather—like the butterfly being transformed within a cocoon—you can embrace the hope of emerging from breast cancer to a beautifully transformed life.

Diagnosis

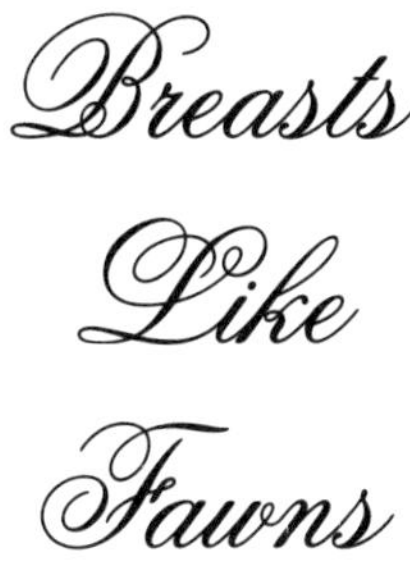

Your two breasts are like the fawns, twins of a gazelle, which feed among the lilies.

—Song of Solomon 4:5

Every woman, I suppose, has her breast story. I don't remember when I first became aware of breasts—my own or anyone else's. I do know that my first nourishment came from my mother's breasts. Between my third and fourteenth birthdays, five siblings were born. Each birth brought a heightened awareness of my mother's breasts as I observed her nursing or using a breast pump. I grew up viewing breasts as a source of physical and emotional sustenance.

By junior high school I observed that the girls in my grade had begun developing breasts. In fact, all the girls in my grade knew whose body was developing what. Our naked bodies were exposed for all to notice and compare during the mandatory showers that brought our physical education classes to an excruciating close. My dread of the clothing- and esteem-stripping showers intensified as the number of girls baring flat chests like mine became fewer and fewer. Thoughts pertaining to my breasts, or more accurately my lack of breasts, were beginning to consume me.

A box of hand-me-down clothes arrived from my beautiful, womanly figured cousin Lois. As I went through the clothes, I noticed several bras. Embarrassed by the obvious disparity between the seemingly large cup size of the bras and the nonexistence of anything on my body to place in such cups, I tucked them toward the back of my underwear drawer.

Guests came to our home that night to visit my parents. Bored, I decided to go to my room and try on one of Lois's bras. There were no push-up wonder bras then; stiff padding was stitched in place within the bra in concentric circles ending at the nipple area in a rather obvious pointy nub. As I put on the bra, I became quite impressed with my instant ample bosom. At last I too had a bustline—in fact, a larger bustline than most of the girls in my grade.

The longer I admired my new image in the mirror, the more I wanted to show it off. I decided to go downstairs and rejoin my family and the visiting couple. Everyone was gathered in the living room watching television—still a fairly new form of entertainment. Soon I became engrossed in the TV show and forgot all about my new look. I lay on my back right smack in front of the TV—placing my elbows out to the sides so I could rest my head on the palms of my hands.

Meanwhile, my toddler brother John was noticing something more interesting than the television—the two pointy mountains that had mysteriously appeared on his sister's chest. Motivated by curiosity, John toddled over and poked his finger into one of the mountains. With a blush erupting and spreading like lava across my cheeks and neck, I looked down. The altered landscape of my chest now consisted of one pointy mountain and one large crater. Wanting to disappear like the top of my collapsed mountain, I slithered towards the upstairs door and made my escape.

Soon after duly venting my anger and humiliation on hapless John, I told my mother that something must be wrong with my body. "Every girl in my grade except me has breasts!" I lamented. What transpired next was a testimony of a mother's pure sacrificial love. During this era of medical care, the fee for an appointment with a doctor came out of the family pocketbook. For most families in our town, that meant a pocketbook that certainly didn't include financing a trip to the doctor for "no good reason."

Nevertheless, there I was in Dr. Johnson's office. My worry overcame my modesty as I timidly shared my distress. Dr. Johnson put down his pen and gave me his full attention as he listened intently. Then he kindly asked, "Sharon, have you ever seen a woman with a child's body?" I thought, then pondered, and finally answered, "No." "Neither have I," Dr. Johnson replied. He concluded my appointment with the reassuring words, "Your body's time-schedule hasn't caught up with the other girls in your grade, but it will. I'm confident your body will begin changing soon. You'll just need to be patient a little longer."

Dr. Johnson was right. During the summer my body changed and I began tenth grade with "two breasts like fawns." They, like the fawns in the Song of Solomon, represented the delicate beauty and promise that precedes full growth. My longed-for breasts were important and special to me. I knew I would never take them for granted.

When I entered college three years later, I was self-conscious about the mole on my face, the beginning of bunions on my feet, the little pouch of extra skin on my tummy, my tendency to slouch, my sparse eyelashes, my blah hair, my weird-shaped nose, my too-long chin, and the possibility of halitosis. Surprisingly, I was content with my breasts. It never occurred to me that my breasts would someday again bring me distress.

Dear God, You did not make a mistake when You created me female nor when You created females with the ability to develop breasts. Your words in the Song of Solomon remind me that—as a gazelle begins as a fawn—a woman begins as a girl. Breasts are likened to two fawns, twins of a gazelle, which feed among

the lilies. Lilies are among the loveliest flowers in Your creation. It is a comfort to know that even when my breasts are a source of distress, they are precious to You, as they are to me. Amen.

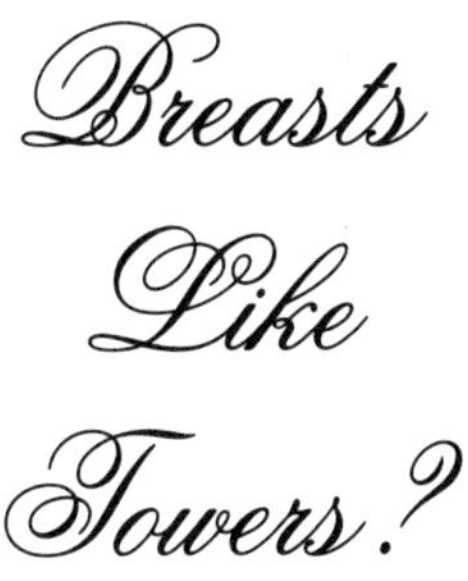

Breasts Like Towers?

I was a wall, and my breasts were like towers.

—Song of Solomon 8:1

I can't help but laugh at the imagery used in the Song of Solomon to depict mature breasts! Towers? In the twenty-first-century rural setting, towers are usually thought of as those structures that hold water or grain and loom distinctly high on the landscape. The exaggeration seems even more pronounced in the cities of today. There I envision towers as skyscrapers soaring into the sky above a skyline of multistoried buildings.

Perhaps, to find meaning in this verse, I need to adjust my notion of towers to the towers of Solomon's day. Maybe at that time, a tower was any structure that significantly protruded from a flat, wall-like background. On the other hand, it's possible that finding a way to describe mature breasts always has been and always will be perplexing!

Somewhere between having "breasts like fawns" and "breasts like towers," a woman matures along with her breasts. Along with maturity comes the realization that her breasts, regardless of their mature size, are an integral part of her femaleness, her uniqueness, her breast story.

My personal breast story evolved during my college years and beyond. My vocabulary expanded far beyond the parameters of first-term Freshman English as I became aware of the myriad of words used for breasts and to describe breasts.

I, along with my peers, realized that our culture places a great deal of emphasis on breasts. The fashion industry and media dictate the ideal woman and set the standard for breasts. Few of us meet the standard, however, as many bewail their "fried egg" breasts while some languish in their state of being over-endowed. Others are willing to invest in breast-enhancing brassieres or cosmetic surgery in an effort to acquire more acceptable breasts. Each of us in our own way is challenged to discover and accept an individual identity as a breasted woman among women.

I was not only a woman among women, however, but also a woman among men. Men are very interested in breasts. At least in our culture, breasts are a source of both visual and tactile stimulation for most men. Breasts are thought of as seductive and sometimes are flaunted to attract and hold the attention of men in general or one or more men in particular. Breasts respond to sexual arousal and are an inherent aspect of a woman's sexuality.

I reserve the pleasure of my breasts for my husband, Colin. I do not equate morality with being prudish. Although I lean toward somewhat conservative dress in public, I delight in wearing feminine and sexy clothes when I'm alone with my husband. Colin enjoys my breasts and I welcome the mutual fulfillment of our sexuality.

The first time I associated my breasts with intense physical pain was shortly after the birth of our first child. As an expectant mother, I envisioned myself snuggling a happy nursing infant to my breasts. Instead, my doctor announced that my nipples were not pronounced enough for my son to suckle. He then handed me artificial nipples resembling bottle nipples and directed me to sterilize them before holding them in place on my breasts.

Within days I developed mastitis, an inflammation of breast tissue. My husband, in graduate school at the time, would arrive home from his night class to find our son wailing with hunger in the crib while I lay in a tub of cool water trying to keep my fever under control until his return. My breasts turned my first two months of motherhood into a painful, frightening episode.

Years later I became aware of an even more threatening breast disease: cancer. I learned about breast self-examination, clinical breast-examination and mammograms. I had difficulty getting into a disciplined routine of monthly breast self-examination, but I was conscientious in scheduling my annual clinical exam and mammogram.

I was being a good girl. I was going by the rules. I felt safe and secure in my belief that bad things didn't happen to good girls who followed the rules. Although imperfect, my body was my friend. Life was good. There were questions that I never thought to ask: "Can a woman be fully female, fully feminine with one breast? With no breasts?"

Dear Creator of breasts, I'm grateful for mature breasts because they are a part of being a woman. I'm also grateful that breasts are but one part of womanhood. Please help me as I continue to discover, define, and accept my identity as a woman. Amen.

Mammograms

And He is the image of the invisible God, the first-born of all creation.
—Colossians 1:15

When and where did I have my first mammogram? Those details of that long-ago experience have been tucked into the recesses of my mind and forgotten. What I do remember, though, is disrobing from the waist up, cleansing away any underarm deodorant or antiperspirant, and putting on a hospital gown—with the opening to the front.

I recall the mammography technician handing me an assortment of mock breasts with hidden lumps of varying sizes. I was to examine the pretend breasts and find the lumps. Most were easy to find, but not all.

Once the technician commenced with the procedure, each of my breasts was in turn sandwiched between flat sections of the mammography machine and compressed. "This may be slightly uncomfortable for just a few seconds," said the technician as she walked to the controls. "Hold your breath," she said, and then, "You can breathe now."

While I waited for the technician to ensure adequate print quality, I read a brochure on breast self-examination. It illustrated the techniques of self-examination, to be completed either while standing or lying down. "Examine your breasts at least monthly," the literature instructed. "Some women find it easiest to remember on the first day of every month, others in conjunction with the menstrual period. Know what your breasts feel like so you can more readily be alerted to any changes." These were the directions I retained.

The technician returned, stated her satisfaction with the clarity of my breast pictures, and permitted me to dress. She handed me an envelope I was to self-address for the mailing of my results. That task done, I was invited to ask any questions. It wasn't until several weeks later that two questions did come to mind: " What do I do if my breasts always feel kind of lumpy?" and "Why isn't there a brochure for husbands on how to examine a wife's breasts?" I suspected most husbands were more familiar with their wives' breasts than the wives were themselves.

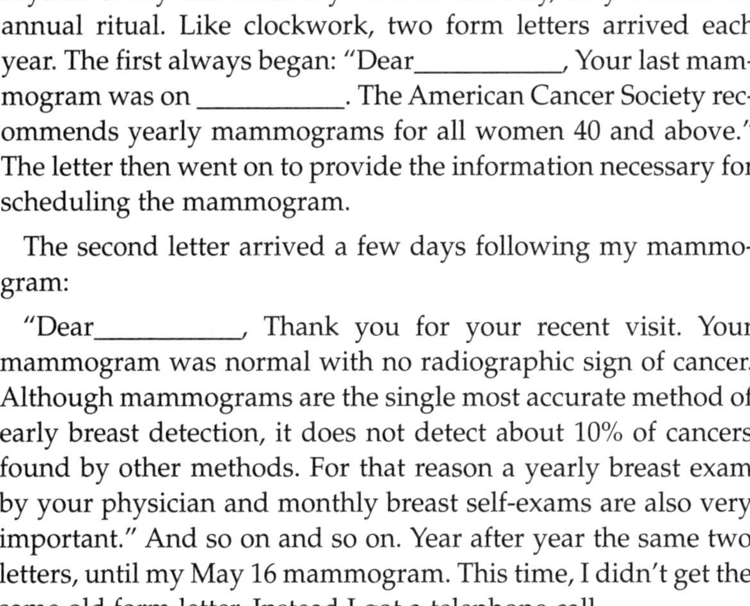

Mammogram appointments became incorporated into the rhythm of my life. After my fortieth birthday, they became an annual ritual. Like clockwork, two form letters arrived each year. The first always began: "Dear___________, Your last mammogram was on ___________. The American Cancer Society recommends yearly mammograms for all women 40 and above." The letter then went on to provide the information necessary for scheduling the mammogram.

The second letter arrived a few days following my mammogram:

"Dear___________, Thank you for your recent visit. Your mammogram was normal with no radiographic sign of cancer. Although mammograms are the single most accurate method of early breast detection, it does not detect about 10% of cancers found by other methods. For that reason a yearly breast exam by your physician and monthly breast self-exams are also very important." And so on and so on. Year after year the same two letters, until my May 16 mammogram. This time, I didn't get the same old form letter. Instead I got a telephone call.

The voice on the telephone was informing me that I needed to schedule an additional mammogram. No, it wouldn't be at the clinic medical-imaging department as before. My May 22 appointment would be at the medical-imaging department of the affiliated hospital. A radiologist would be available to read my mammogram.

The voice didn't sound alarmed or particularly concerned. "It's just an extra precaution," I reasoned. "Perhaps this is a new procedure." Yes, mammograms were still rather routine and ho-hum . . . but not quite as ho-hum as they had been before the out-of-routine telephone call.

Dear Creator, I don't comprehend medical imaging. Neither do I understand how a mammography machine can make images of my breast that reveal what is otherwise invisible. Perhaps for now comprehension and understanding are less important than believing. I believe Your word in Colossians 1:15 that calls Christ "the image of the invisible God, the first-born of all creation." Help me to place my faith in You, the invisible God to Whom all things are visible, and in the supremacy of Christ, Your image. Amen.

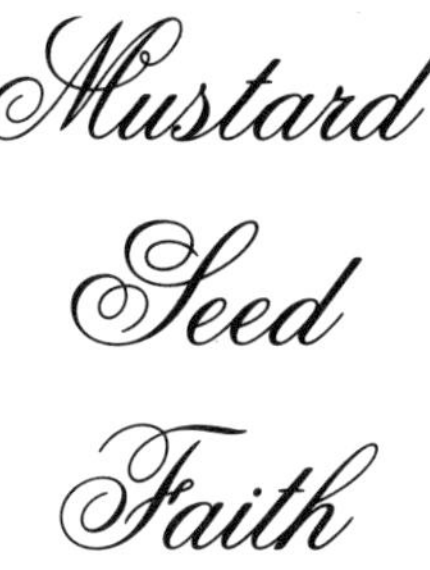

Mustard Seed Faith

Consider what a great forest is set on fire by a small spark.

—*James* 3:5 (NIV)

"I tell you the truth, if you have faith as small as a mustard seed, you can say to this mountain, 'Move from here to there' and it will move. Nothing will be impossible for you."

—*Matthew* 17:20-21 (NIV)

I narrowed my eyes to a squint and studied the suspicious spot of white on the grey breast. The hospital radiologist had clipped my mammography image into place on the lit screen and pointed to the spot that had necessitated a second mammogram appointment. "It looks like it's approximately one centimeter—the size of a small pea," he said. So small, yet so foreboding. "Your primary physician will refer you for a biopsy," he concluded, turning off the machine.

Driving home, my mind fixates on small things. It seems paradoxical to me: How could small things hold great power? Have deadly potential?

I think of James 3:5, referring to the admonition to control one's tongue. The verse likens the tongue to a small spark capable of setting a great forest on fire. How true, I concede, as I contemplate the power of one's tongue. A lie, an angry rebuke, a harsh criticism, gossip—all carry the potential to slander, betray, corrupt, estrange, wound, and destroy.

I recall spring 1984. Serving as short-term missionaries in Japan, my husband, children, and I took a train trip during the school break to visit the home of one of our dormitory daughters. Her father, a seven-year-old boy at the time of the bombing of Hiroshima, had survived and gone on to become a Christian missionary. The train took us through Hiroshima and into Nagasaki. I'll never forget the evidence of nuclear destruction I observed at the Nagasaki museum commemorating the bombing. An atom is such a small part of matter. Yet an atomic bomb holds the power to annihilate cities.

My thoughts continue to ramble. A small indiscretion can destroy trust, a relationship, a marriage, a family. One crime can ruin a reputation and cause a forfeiture of freedom. One small malignant tumor can metastasize and ravage, even kill, a human body. I am gripped with fear as I remember the small, barely visible, harmless-looking spot I saw minutes ago.

The Holy Spirit, so much more powerful than destructive small things and fear, is now bringing another thought to my reeling mind. It is a mustard-seed thought. I recall Jesus' words, "I tell you the truth, if you have faith as small as a mustard seed, you can say to this mountain, 'move from here to there,' and it will move. Nothing will be impossible to you."

Pulling in our driveway and walking indoors, I am eager to find something in my home. I walk to the kitchen cabinet and rummage through my spice containers, excitement and faith mounting. There it is, among my pickling spices—a jar of mustard seeds! I remove one of the yellow seeds and study it. It is small. I decide I am able to exercise faith the size of this small mustard seed. Fetching my Bible and a roll of transparent tape,

I symbolically tape the mustard seed to the inside cover of the Bible.

Whether my mountain is a small malignant tumor capable of destroying my body or a small fear able to consume my peace of mind, I claim faith to overcome. Nothing will be impossible!

My omnipotent God, I am thankful for the parable of mustard-seed faith. Jesus knew that at times faith would seem too small for big problems. I'm so grateful He chose something small like a mustard seed to help encourage faith. I am able to have faith the size of a mustard seed. Because nothing is impossible for You, I can bring my mustard-seed-small faith to You and believe that nothing is impossible for me. In Jesus' name I pray. Amen.

Where is Number Twelve? Discharge Instructions Following Breast Biopsy

Lead me in Thy truth and teach me,
for thou art the God of my salvation;
For thee I wait all the day.
—Psalm 25:5

The day was June 12. As I drove alone to the hospital for an ultrasound guided-needle biopsy, my mind meandered back to a similar day two years earlier.

My annual mammogram then had revealed a suspicious spot on my left breast. My primary physician scheduled me for a breast biopsy. She had taken time to explain the procedure. She hadn't seemed particularly concerned, so I had followed her cue and not been alarmed. During the five-day wait for that appointment, my husband and I had maintained a light, positive attitude. We had decided to keep the scheduled biopsy to ourselves and privately addressed the situation in prayer.

Two nights before that biopsy, however, I awoke in a cold sweat and was pierced by the realization, "I could die of breast cancer!" My predawn thoughts ran rampant through an ever-escalating disastrous scenario. Relieved when my husband finally stirred, I burst into sobs and blurted out my thoughts and fears. His words of comfort and prayer consoled my fright, but we both began to take the upcoming biopsy more seriously.

Though he had been in a busy time at work, my husband had taken a portion of the day off to join me at the hospital for the biopsy. The procedure was almost painless and seemed quite minor. Thinking back now, I could not recall my feelings nor the duration between the biopsy and my follow-up appointment; I only remembered hearing "Good news! It was just calcified cells—nothing to be concerned about." The whole episode had left me feeling relieved and concluding that a biopsy isn't such a big deal after all.

⁂

Heavy traffic jolted me back to the present day and the recognition that I was now in a driving situation that demanded my undivided attention. Once parked in the hospital lot, I again mentally reviewed the words I anticipated hearing at my upcoming biopsy follow-up appointment: "Good news! It's just calcified cells again—this time in your right breast." Both my husband and I were so upbeat that we had agreed it wouldn't be necessary for him to accompany me to this biopsy.

The Breast Center was more attractively decorated than I remembered. Technology had advanced in two years. The ultrasound guided technique was even less uncomfortable than my previous procedure. Leaving the Breast Center, I felt the experience had been as positive as possible. Even the concluding words were assuring: "We make every effort to have the results to your primary physician within twenty-four hours. If your physician hasn't contacted you by 4:30 tomorrow afternoon, give her a call."

"Being an experienced biopsy patient has its merits," I smugly acknowledged. This time I had been proactive in planning a treat for myself on the way home—a bit of paradise in the form of a close-out sale at a large garden center. Because I had just left a hospital, I even took advantage of the opportunity to request help transporting my bountiful bargains to the car. As I drove the "conservatory-mobile" into our driveway, all my husband could identify was my sunny face smiling through the foliage and blossoms.

Before bedtime, I reviewed the take-home handout entitled "Discharge Instructions Following Breast Biopsy." There were eleven of them—a seemingly complete list that included everything from diet recommendations and bra-wearing guidelines to Steri-Strips and constipation.

Reflecting upon the events of the day, I checked the time—9:30 P.M. Nineteen hours to go until 4:30 P.M., when I would find out the biopsy results. "How do I get through the next nineteen hours?" I wondered, as my upbeat, sunny-smile attitude waned and a troublesome uneasiness set in. There should be a twelfth instruction that would answer the question, "What do you do with your mind during the twenty-four hours between having a breast biopsy and finding out the results?"

Dear God, I'm so grateful that Your instructions in the Bible are given to lead and to teach during every need—even following a breast biopsy. I pray for a biopsy report that contains truth. Thank You for being the God of my salvation regardless of the biopsy outcome. Thank You for being with me moment by moment as I wait "all the day." Amen.

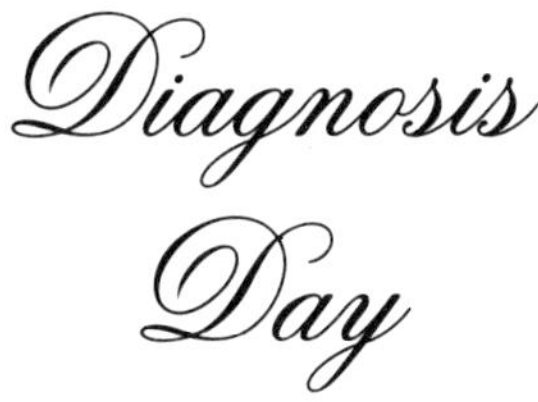

Diagnosis Day

A gentle answer turns away wrath, but a harsh word stirs up anger. The tongue of the wise makes knowledge acceptable, but the mouth of fools sprouts folly.

—Proverbs 15:1,2

It was a long afternoon, that thirteenth day of June—the day following my breast biopsy. I busied myself pulling weeds in the flower gardens until late afternoon; then showered in preparation for the anticipated telephone call.

Time, along with my body, had dragged through the day—a day so routine, yet anything but routine. Though I anticipated good news, waiting for the biopsy results was taking its toll.

4:30, 4:31, 4:32. No telephone call. I recited to myself the exact words spoken to me yesterday as I left the breast center: "If your physician hasn't contacted you by 4:30 tomorrow afternoon, give her a call."

Reaching for the telephone, I felt like a lady holding on to a trapeze. For the moment, I was poised on a safe perch; but now, as I dialed the clinic, I was taking the step forward that would ultimately lead to either exhilaration or a fall into the unknown.

"I don't think your physician has received your biopsy results yet, but I'll check and get back to you," the voice at the clinic answered in response to my inquiry.

First a day of hours that passed in slow motion, then minutes that crawled, and now seconds measured by my pounding heartbeat. Startled by the ring of the telephone, I grabbed the receiver. "Your results just arrived. Your doctor will see you after her last appointment. Can you be here by 5:30?" "Yes . . . . Should I bring my husband?" I was fishing. My mind strained as I listened for hidden meaning in her response, "I don't think it's necessary for him to come." "Ah-ha! That must mean everything is fine," I cautiously concluded.

With the clinic a thirty-minute drive away, I quickly changed clothes and sought out my husband. Hearing him with our young-adult son in the basement, I yelled down the steps, "I'm on my way to the clinic. I guess you don't need to come. I'll be back soon."

Alone in the waiting room, I was immediately summoned to a seat in an examining room. Noticing a prenatal magazine, I thumbed through to the page that described fetal development at seven months. I was trying to imagine the fetus in my daughter's womb resembling the illustration when my physician and a young woman entered. I pointed to the picture and shared, "That's how my first grandchild looks now."

We weren't there for chit-chat, however. After introducing me to her intern, my physician responded to the question asked by my demeanor. Always warm and friendly, she gently relayed her difficult answer, "I'm so sorry, but you do have breast cancer."

I felt nurtured despite the news that crushed my hope. I studied her face and was touched by her genuine concern, her caring, her direct yet sensitive eye contact. Glancing at the intern, I caught an expression that belied her intended professionalism. It was a look of curiosity, of wondering, "How is this woman going to react?"

Well . . . how was I reacting? Caught off guard for sure! I really had expected to hear, "Good news! It's only calcified cells again!" I was being given the courtesy of a few moments of silence to absorb the surprising news. I sighed deeply, realizing that I felt okay—almost serene.

My physician, an astute reader of body language, perceived mine to be communicating, "What now?" Methodically and thoroughly, she obliged, as though I was her only patient of the day. In fact, I suspected this popular doctor was probably exhausted after a day filled with numerous needy patients. Yet there was no peeking at the clock, no hurrying me out the door.

Her gentle response to my need softened the stark reality of my situation and enabled me to accept her knowledge. She concluded her explanation of the next steps with, "Call the surgeon tomorrow to schedule your consultation for next week." Then, noting the magazine still open across my lap, she smiled and confidently exclaimed, "And you'll be just fine when that baby comes!"

Dear Lord, It's been a long, tedious, disappointing day. I did not receive the answer I hoped for. I have barely begun processing the news I received. But I am thankful for my physician's gentle manner and the truth found in Proverbs 15:2. The tongue of the wise helps make even unacceptable knowledge acceptable. Amen.

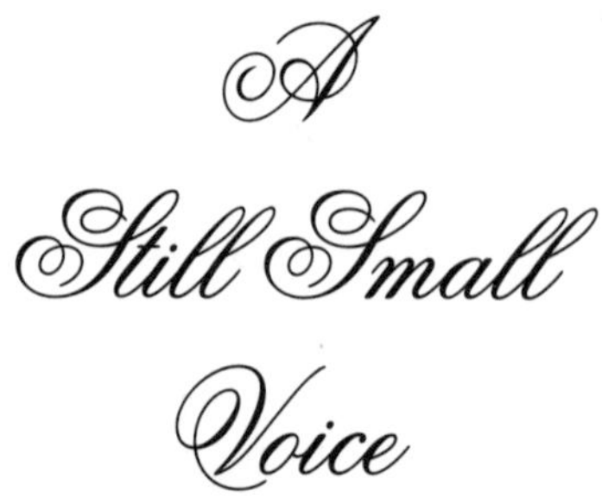

And he said, "Go forth, and stand on the mount before the Lord." And behold, the Lord passed by, and a great and strong wind rent the mountains, and broke in pieces the rocks before the Lord, but the Lord was not in the wind; and after the wind an earthquake, but the Lord was not in the earthquake; and after the earthquake a fire, but the Lord was not in the fire; and after the fire a still small voice.

—1 Kings 19:11,12

Jarred out of my whirlwind of thoughts by the realization that I was driving too fast, I looked at the speedometer: 75 miles per hour—and the posted speed limit was 60! I was thankful I hadn't been pulled over for speeding. What would I have told the law enforcement officer? "I'm driving under the influence of breast cancer"?

Though I stayed calm and clear-headed as my physician informed me of my breast cancer diagnosis, once in the car, my thoughts began to spin. When I became aware of my speeding, I scanned the area around me. I had driven over half the twenty-five miles to home oblivious to my surroundings. "You've got to concentrate on driving home safely," I scolded myself as I turned on the radio. I needed to focus on something, anything other than my situation.

The radio was already set on the Christian station I often listened to while driving. A nationally acclaimed pastor was expounding on the topic of trust. A scramble of dizzying thoughts was racing through my mind: How can I tell Colin? He should have been with me. He'll be disappointed that he wasn't with me. When I had asked the caller from the clinic if my husband should come, she had replied, "I don't think that will be necessary." From her response, I had assumed that my husband didn't need to come because the report was good news. The result of my mistaken assumption was a double whammy—the report was not good news. And my husband should have been included in the receiving of it.

Now, the radio program was offering the perfect anecdote for my state of mind. "Trust . . ." continued the speaker on the radio. This messenger from God was speaking on the very topic I needed at the very time I needed it. I was unable to focus on the details of his message; only the word trust was able to take root and remain securely in my mind. That one word was able to quiet my inner storm and I was able to be sufficiently calmed and comforted to grasp the concluding words of his message, "We can trust God regardless of the challenges we encounter in life."

The program concluded; the top of the news was to be announced next. I turned off the radio, loathing the idea of any more news of any kind. Then during those few moments between turning off the radio and allowing my scattered thoughts to focus, I realized that two clear messages had lodged in my mind. The first was: You can trust Me though this. The second: This will not be a wasted time in your life.

I knew beyond any doubt that the origin of the two thoughts was God. In the midst of my storm, I had been given the gift of a holy revelation. I was glad I was still a few miles from home. I needed to bask in, to savor, to absorb what had just transpired.

I recalled a once-confusing Old Testament Scripture passage. Elijah went before God with a need and requested an answer. When the Lord passed by there was a strong wind, an earthquake, and a fire—but Elijah did not hear God's voice in any of these powerful, frightening events. Then God spoke—in a still small voice.

The revelation became clear to me: in the midst of powerful, frightening events, God is able to speak to us personally in a still small voice. I realized I wouldn't be spared my own version of wind, earthquake, and fire; but I could trust God to quietly speak to me. As I turned into our driveway, I was thinking, "Whatever happens from this moment on, I know where I must go when I begin to feel overwhelmed. I must find a quiet place where I can wait with expectancy to again hear God's still small voice."

Almighty God, who spoke to Elijah so many centuries ago, I'm grateful that You continue to speak to Your children today. You, who could speak through wind, earthquake, and fire, choose to often speak in a quiet voice. Please help calm my inner storm so I can hear and follow Your voice. Amen.

Telling, Learning, Deciding, Waiting

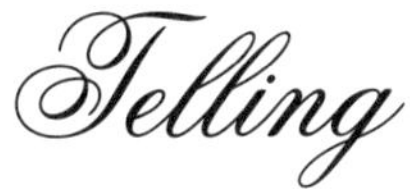

How lovely on the mountains are the feet of him who brings good news.
—Isaiah 52:7

Everyone, it seems, is happy to bring good news. But what about bad news? I found that there never is a good time for bad news. No one wants to bring bad news; no one wants to hear bad news—ever.

My husband, Colin, was the first to hear my bad news after the breast cancer diagnosis. He and our young adult son Matt were in a room watching television when I returned home from the physician's office. I asked my husband if we could change our supper plans—if, instead of the stir-fry meal I had planned to prepare, Matt could telephone for an order of delivery pizza. With that practicality out of the way, I casually invited my husband to join me in our bedroom.

Colin took the news hard. He sat on the edge of our bed and sobbed—great, deep sobs from the depth of his being. He, too, had expected good news. He was unprepared for my anything-but-good news. He was clearly devastated. I had never before seen my husband in such unrestrained sadness—not even when he had lost his brother, or his father.

Colin and I would be celebrating our thirty-third wedding anniversary soon; yet I suddenly felt as shy and awkward as I had on our first date. I sensed that there was now an intruder in our bedroom, in our marriage. My bad news had brought into our intimate relationship an unwelcome trespasser—breast cancer.

I sat on the bed beside my husband and we embraced. I wanted to cry with him, but I couldn't. Why hadn't I cried yet?

For now, I could only receive his tears as my own. I ached with the awareness that my bad news was capable of bringing pain and distress to those I loved. After the tears came his many questions, followed by my few answers, followed by the realization of our need to tell Matt, followed by the arrival of the pizza deliverer.

The pizza, thin-crust pepperoni with onions and green olives—our favorite celebration food—was a contradiction to this grim day. The pizza failed in its usual power to seduce and satisfy our senses. Instead, it tasted like the cardboard box it was delivered in. Managing somehow to chew and swallow without saliva, I was relieved to be temporarily diverted by the television show and Matt's enjoyment of the delivered treat.

The meal finished, the television was turned off. I faced Matt and began, "You probably are figuring out that something is happening . . ." Matt, in his youthful optimism and faith, seemed to receive the news well. "God will help and it will turn out okay," he assured us, and he accepted our request to keep the news within our household for the time being.

Following our consultation with the surgeon, the surgery date was set. We would have a five-week delay due to the back-to-back two-week vacations of my two surgeons. Yes, five weeks was an unusually long waiting period, but we were assured it was nothing to be concerned about.

The first of many difficulties prompted by the long biding was answering the "telling" questions. Who do we tell sooner to gain support and who do we tell later to spare excess worry? When should we tell our other adult children? My mother and siblings? My in-laws? Our pastor? Our friends?

Would it have been easier if the surgery had been scheduled within a week, sparing us the painstaking "best possible time and place" telling decisions? Regardless of timeline, could I have done a better job of telling my bad news? Perhaps so. Perhaps not. I don't know.

I do know that I prayed about whom to tell, how to tell, and when to tell. I do believe that God heard and answered my prayers. I do recognize that no two people received and responded to my news in the same way. I do understand that there are times to bring mountain-top good news; but there are also times to bring valley-bottom bad news. I do accept the reality that I did the best I could in my telling.

Dear God, it is You who brought Your angel to the frightened shepherds to proclaim, "Do not be afraid; for behold, I bring you good news of great joy which shall be for all people; for today in the city of David there has been born for you a Savior, who is Christ the Lord." I'm so grateful that Your bringing the ultimate good news—the Savior, Christ the Lord—transcends the experiencing and telling of my bad news. Amen.

Naive or Prudent?

The naive inherit folly, but the prudent are crowned with knowledge.

—*Proverbs 14:18*

Grace and peace be multiplied to you in the knowledge of God and of Jesus our Lord; seeing that His divine power has granted to us everything pertaining to life and godliness, through the true knowledge of Him who called us by His own glory and excellence.

—*II Peter 1:2,3*

I must admit, however reluctantly, that I was a bit naive when it came to cancer jargon. Oh, I was familiar with the basic "big C" vocabulary that has become all too common in newspaper and magazine articles. But, my knowledge of cancer-related words was limited to gleanings from the media and conversations with people touched in some way by the disease.

Proverbs 14:18 warns that the naive inherit folly. My dictionary defines *folly* as behavior arising from stupidity; misguided behavior liable to end disastrously. With my health, my future well-being and that of my family, and perhaps even my life at stake, I realize that remaining naive is no longer an option.

Scanning the "P" segment of the dictionary, my index finger follows my eyes down the column to the word *prudent*. I want to know the exact definition and find it to be "foresight leading a person to avoid error or danger." I am a person needing to avoid error or danger. I need to be a prudent person crowned with knowledge about breast cancer.

I need to gain knowledge and I need to gain it immediately. Forcing my will to prevail over my frayed emotions, I find the folder containing the breast cancer information I have received so far and gaze at it in numb silence. I feel like a scared little girl confronted prematurely with the task of learning the alphabet. My new A-B-C alphabet begins: About Breast Cancer.

Opening the folder, the top page is a copy of my breast biopsy report. My reading soon becomes bogged down in a quicksand of unfamiliar words. Ultrasound-guided core needle biopsy, right breast lesion, asymmetric density, oblique view, hypoechoic area, localized sonographically, prepped with Bentodine, lidocaine, epinephrine, sodium biocarbonate. Through my sluggish mind a new concern surfaces: "Will I be able to grasp the knowledge I need in order to be prudent?"

I swallow my pride and turn to the second page, entitled "Core Breast Biopsy—Pathology Report." It is from the chief of breast imaging—a rather unique job title, I grimly muse. More new words along with a profusion of measurement terms and numbers assault my intellect. Staging parameters, histological type, Nottingham score. My mind begins to spin as my confidence in understanding the report diminishes.

I page through one of the several breast cancer-related booklets I've received and find a glossary. Adjuvant therapy, ductal carcinoma, estrogen-receptor assay, invasive, noninvasive, lobular carcinoma, lymphedema, metastasis, modified radical mastectomy, myocutaneous flap, neoadjuvant therapy, prosthesis, recurrence, reconstructive surgery, segmental mastectomy . . .

and on and on. I feel as though some sadistic villain has enrolled me in a medical school oncology class against my will.

Discouraged, I thumb through the other booklets. More perplexing words, numbers and measurements, diagrams and photographs of breasts—breasts with cancer. I don't want to know these words and numbers and their perilous meanings. I don't want to see these diagrams and pictures. I don't want to meet with the surgeon. I don't want to deal with any of this.

Then I remember the word *prudent*. Whether I *want* to learn about breast cancer or not isn't the issue. I *must* gain knowledge about breast cancer and I must do so quickly. There will be decisions to make and they must be made soon. But how can my mind be prudent when my heart wants to cling to innocent naivety?

I feel exposed—physically, emotionally, and intellectually inadequate for the demands before me. I feel like a woman quivering in the corner, crowned with a dunce cap. A confident prudent woman crowned with knowledge? Where do I even begin?

Downcast, I reach for another book of words—the Bible—and flip through it until I stop at II Peter. My eyes are drawn to chapter 1, verses 2 and 3—God has given me His answer. I will begin my quest for knowledge about what I do not know with my knowledge of who I do know—God and Jesus my Lord.

Dear God and Jesus my Lord, I believe that Your divine power has granted me everything pertaining to life and godliness. I ask that Your grace and peace be multiplied in me as I seek to be a prudent woman crowned with knowledge. Amen.

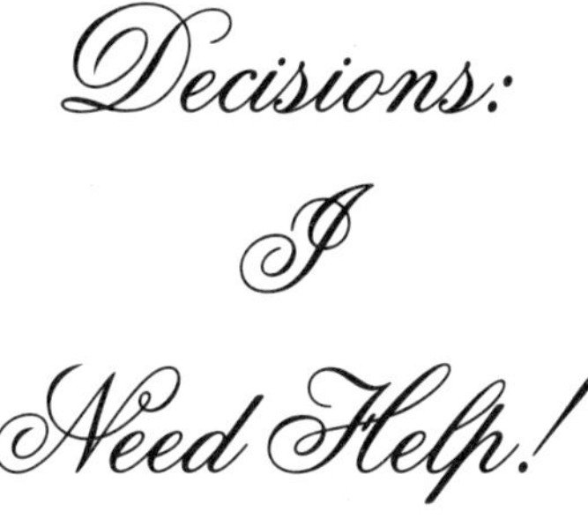

Decisions: I Need Help!

Make me know Thy ways, O Lord;
Teach me Thy paths.

—Psalm 25:4

Trust in the Lord with all your heart, And do not lean on your own understanding. In all your ways acknowledge Him, And He will make your paths straight.

—Proverbs 3:5,6

It is the day after my diagnosis. I'm thankful it is a Wednesday—the day I attend a weekly intercessory prayer group. This morning I tell the small group of women my news and allow myself to fall into their safety net of love, caring, and prayer support.

Uplifted and strengthened, I return home to my husband and his news. My primary physician had come in on her day off to telephone my husband and inquire about his and my well-being. She also had met with the surgeon. Upon learning that today would be his final day at the office prior to a two-week vacation, she has scheduled our appointment with him for mid-afternoon. Decisions need to be made. We are advised to look through the materials already received.

I'd looked over the materials last night and hadn't understood the words. How can I—how can my husband and I—make decisions based on words we don't understand? How can we be expected to master Breast Cancer 101 in a few hours—hours clouded by shock, denial, and anxiety? The peace I was enveloped in during the prayer group is wavering as I succumb to the realization that my husband and I will inevitably be unprepared when we meet with the surgeon.

The clock—not my appetite—tells me it's time for lunch. I need to decide on something simple to prepare for our meal. I stare blankly into the cabinet, then the refrigerator. Nothing appeals to me. Every option seems like too much effort. I force my scattered brain cells to focus on the seemingly momentous decision at hand: ham, tuna salad, or a bacon-lettuce-tomato sandwich. Somehow I manage to place slices of ham between slices of bread for each of us, count out two bananas, and pour two glasses of milk.

My mind swirls as my husband and I choke down our third tasteless meal. "How do saliva and taste buds know to shut down during times like these?" I ask, probing for light conversation. Neither of us is up to talking, though. Just concentrating on our need to remain nourished is draining enough. Bite, chew thoroughly, sip, swallow—repeat until plate and glass are empty.

Clearing the table, I am unable to decide whether to rinse our plates and glasses before placing them in the dishwasher. Should I bring the banana peels to the garden compost pile now or wait until we get back? What does one wear to a consultation appointment with a breast-cancer surgeon? Should we leave a note for our son, Matt? Should we leave the air conditioner on, or turn it off? What about our supper? These immediate decisions seem overwhelming to me. How can I be expected to make life-altering decisions when I can't even decide the basic and mundane?

I feel like I've been reduced to a mechanical robot, programmed by years of practice to proceed through well-rehearsed decision-making motions. But . . . I've never rehearsed making breast cancer surgery decisions. Help!

O Lord, I need Your help. I simply don't know enough to make the decisions that need to be made. I can't even decide which words I should use to pray, so I will pray with Your words. Please help me know the way I should go and teach me Your choice of path. I choose to trust in You with all my heart and lean not on my own understanding. I acknowledge You in all my ways and ask You to make my paths straight. Amen.

Mountains

I will lift up my eyes to the mountains; from whence shall my help come? My help comes from the Lord, Who made heaven and earth.

—Psalm 121:1,2

"One is a fool who does not climb Mt. Fuji once, but one is a greater fool who climbs Mt. Fuji twice." Those were the words of a familiar Japanese saying that echoed in my ears that August evening in 1984, when my husband, sister, brother-in-law, and I began our ascent up Japan's Mt. Fuji. We had been told that many of the Japanese place significance in worshipping at the Shinto shrine at Mt. Fuji's summit before they die—believing that its high altitude brings them closest to the gods.

Halfway through our two-year stint as short-term missionaries at the Christian Academy in Japan, my husband and I were elated to receive the letter from my sister Janet informing us that she and her husband would be visiting us in August.

"August is the best month to climb Mt. Fuji," prompted career missionaries who had already made the trek. Mt. Fuji—Japan's highest mountain, the magnificent snow-capped jewel we had often admired in art works and travelogues—was beckoning us to its summit. Would our guests be interested in joining us on the adventure? Our inquiry to Janet and Keith and their affirmative response flashed across the Pacific Ocean like lightening. The four of us would climb Mt. Fuji!

Soon the day of our climb arrived, and we found ourselves among a gaggle of Japanese hikers snaking our way up the lava-rock mountainside. The plan was to embark on the climb in the early evening, ascend throughout the night, and reach the summit around five o'clock in the morning—just in time to see the sunrise from the highest point in the Land of the Rising Sun.

The adrenaline-powered take off at Station One just above the timberline gradually fizzled as the realities of fatigue, sore feet, and hunger set in. Layers of protective clothing were transferred item by item from bulging backpacks to bewildered bodies as first summer, then autumn, and finally winter temperatures engulfed us. The rigorous climb was assaulting my body and soul.

Chatter among the Japanese dwindled to a single word of camaraderie that even we could understand and utter—*gambate* (persevere). The progression became an endurance test, a countdown of time, steps, whispers of breath. Exhausted, I was concluding, "One is a fool who climbs Mt. Fuji at all!" I began to question my ability to complete the climb.

After hours of being fixated on the path before my feet, I raised my head to look around me. What met my eyes, from this mountain observatory, was the most amazing panorama of nighttime splendor I had ever seen. The vastness of the heavens, the moon, and the stars met the expanse of the village-lit earth—an all-encompassing black velvet cloak studded with sparkling diamonds. From my vantage point, the heavens were indistinguishable from the earth—it was all God's seamless creation. Gazing in wonder at the overwhelming beauty surrounding me, I recalled the words that introduce Psalm 121: "I will lift up my eyes to the mountains."

Refreshed and energized, I surveyed the expanse of mountain looming before me. I looked to my Lord Who made heaven and earth to help me complete the climb. As we zigzagged ever upward to nourishment-providing Stations Seven, Eight, and Nine, the thinning air began to make us giddy. We paid the few yen that entitled us to a small resting space among dozens of other climbers—but the assorted noises emerging from our dozing comrades drove us to unrestrained guffaws instead of our much-needed snooze.

We arrived at Station Ten—the summit—just in time to look to the eastern horizon and witness the rising of the sun—right on schedule, as ordained by its Divine Maker. Hunger and fatigue faded away with the night. Awestruck, I was transfixed on the prize awaiting us victorious climbers—the brilliant fuchsia-colored sun, veiled by wisps of morning's mist, ushering in the dawn of a new day.

* * *

Today I am at home in my own country. Another mountain is before me. Unlike Mt. Fuji, this is a mountain I have not chosen to climb, and—like the Japanese—I will never want to climb this mountain twice. I have just begun climbing its foreign course, ascending to a different summit. My mountain is breast cancer; my course is its treatment; the name of my summit is optimal health.

The progression up this mountain, too, will have many stations. The obvious stations will be the various treatment settings, each with its own offerings. The less obvious stations will be spiritual, emotional, and relational in nature. I will likely become exhausted, depleted, and discouraged. As in my climb up Mt. Fuji, there will be times I will question my ability to continue.

I don't know all that I will encounter along the way. I don't know what I'll find at the summit. I don't know if the climb will be worth it—but I do know the One who does. I will be able to look behind and ahead and above and know that His presence is surrounding me. I will proceed knowing that God will help me and guide me to my summit. Perhaps at this summit, I will again be rewarded for my climb—awestruck by the dawning of a new day.

> **O Lord, regardless of the nature of my mountain that looms ahead, I need only to look beyond it to be reminded of You. You create and ordain; You are in control of time and space and all that exists—yet You are willing to heed my calls for help. I choose to keep my eyes on You as I climb my mountain. Amen.**

Changes

Jesus Christ is the same yesterday and today, yes and forever.

—Hebrews 13:8

Sitting on the sofa, I gazed out the living room window and sighed. Less than two weeks ago, energy and ideas had surged through my body and mind as I visualized a summer filled with entertaining, with redesigning and expanding flower beds, and with freezing fresh produce. Now I was caught in limbo between a sense of urgency nagging me to complete planned projects before my surgery, and lethargy as I coveted time to simply process what was happening to me. Nearly all plans for the summer would need to be changed—either postponed or modified.

As I gazed at the animal life around me, a hummingbird caught my eye, then other birds and a butterfly. They all looked so healthy and content, going about their daily routine. Like it or not, ready or not, my daily routine would be changing. In the past, I had prided myself on adapting unusually well to change . . . but to this change?

Scheduled surgery was still weeks away, but I was finding it difficult to focus on anything but the fact that a malignant tumor was in my breast. While I mechanically worked my way through the first few items on my must-do-before-surgery list, my almost-constant awareness of the intact tumor was robbing me of zeal. How could I focus on the joy of living during the days ahead instead of on the impending changes and on the tumor?

From my vantage point on the sofa, I noticed the kaleidoscope I had made several years ago and given to my husband on his birthday. We both had taken pleasure in this personalized tubular viewing devise, created especially for him. I recalled selecting, from the bounty of items provided by the class instructor, fragments of colorful glass and paper and several tiny items depicting Colin's personal talents, interests, and hobbies.

Though my husband and I had found the kaleidoscope enchanting for a few days, it soon lost its novelty and was placed on a shelf. Over the years, the kaleidoscope had become nothing more than an interesting, but never used, home accent piece.

Somehow, I felt drawn to it today. I pulled myself from the sofa, walked across the room, and lifted the kaleidoscope from its cradle. Giving it a bit of a turn toward the sun, I raised it to my eye. I was amazed at the pattern magnified through the angled mirrors—a design of twelve clusters, each with six distinct crosses, was prominent on a backdrop of reds, greens, and gold. I'd forgotten that I had included a small cross while assembling the kaleidoscope. It was as though God was creating a miniature stained-glass window especially for me.

Though I hadn't prayed, God heard my heart's cry—my need to establish a changeless focus in my mind and life. He provided His perfect answer in this amazing way.

The cross was to be my focus today and every day throughout this summer and beyond. True, there would be changes ahead. Because I was moving into such unfamiliar territory, I couldn't even fathom all of the changes before me. That's why God was drawing my focus to the cross, to Jesus Christ—the One who is changeless in the midst of change.

I lingered on the visual image before my eye, then rotated the instrument to enjoy a myriad of other intricate patterns. After several minutes and dozens of images had passed, I tried once again to view a design with crosses. I rotated and turned and even shook the kaleidoscope, but was unable to create another cross pattern. I finally gave up and put the kaleidoscope away.

* * *

As I experience the changes ahead, sometimes Jesus will be in view and at other times He will be obscured. Yet, just as I know that the cross remains in the kaleidoscope, even when I am unable to bring it into view, I also know that Jesus remains in my life. He is and will remain my focus, my constant, throughout the changes in my body and life. I am able to move on with my changing life because of my confidence that He never changes.

> **Jesus Christ, I acknowledge You as my Savior and Lord. Please help me during this time of change to keep my focus on You. I believe You are with me always. I'm so grateful that You are "the same yesterday and today, yes and forever." Amen.**

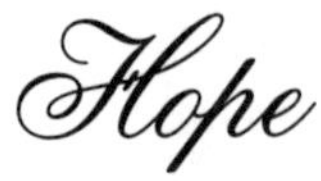

For in hope we have been saved, but hope that is seen is not hope; for why does one also hope for what one sees? But if we hope for what we do not see, with perseverance we wait eagerly for it.

—Romans 8:24,25

Today my sister Carol gave me a gift—a stuffed animal from the Beanie Babies collection. The little honey-colored bear is in a kneeling position with its paws folded in prayer. Upon reading the attached heart-shaped red tag, I discover that my bear even has a name and birth date. My new furry praying friend's name? "Hope."

Though it is just an inanimate object, I realize I need this little bear to be my visual reminder of hope during the months ahead. Hope finds a new home among the other gifts I've received—flowering plants and an array of greeting cards. Hope and her entourage serve to remind me of the many people who care and are praying for me. In a sense, the praying bear, vibrant blossoms, and cheery cards are all messengers of hope.

Glancing at my new little Hope, I realize she looks very much like a storybook bear. My mind drifts and I begin musing about my own life story. I have just begun to live the chapter on my breast cancer experience.

What am I hoping for in this chapter of my life? I hope for a successful treatment plan. I hope for healing. Ultimately, I hope my life story proceeds with my being healthy again, returning to a normal life, and "living happily ever after" free of cancer.

If only I could peek ahead through my life storybook to the last page to ensure that my hopes will be fulfilled. Then I could live my breast cancer chapter with confidence and peace of mind.

But now I recall, "hope that is seen is not hope," and that hope isn't real if we already know the outcome. My breast cancer experience is not a chapter in a storybook that can be read ahead. No, instead I must live my cancer story day by day with living hope. As recorded in Romans 8:25, I am given the gift of hoping for what I do not see, and with perseverance I will wait eagerly for it.

Dear Lord of hope, You alone know how my life story will unfold from this day forward. You also know my hopes for the future. I thank You for your gift of hope and for the encouragement my little "Hope" bear brings. I ask You for perseverance sufficient for each day. As I place my trust in You, help me to wait with eagerness for what I do not see. Amen.

Patience

Be patient . . . Behold, the farmer waits for the precious produce of the soil, being patient about it, until it gets the early and late rains. You too be patient; strengthen your hearts, for the coming of the Lord is at hand.

—James 5:7,8

My patience was being stretched and tested. Over the years, friends and colleagues had often complimented me on my patience. True, I was patient in my interactions with people.

Patience has more than one dimension, however. For me, it now meant the ability to wait, to persevere, without being consumed by debilitating thoughts. Like the fable of the tortoise and the hare, my mind was racing like a hare to the finish line of my course of treatment—while the calendar trudged on toward the first phase. Regardless of my patience or lack thereof, there remained twenty-four hours in each day.

Five weeks between diagnosis and surgery was certainly not the norm. The abnormality occurred because the recommended duo of surgeons—my primary surgeon and a surgeon experienced with the sentinel lymph node procedure—had scheduled back-to-back two-week vacations. Our options were: wait or change surgeons. My husband and I had opted to wait. But . . . that had been before I realized the challenge of waiting would be greater than my patience to endure the wait.

⁂

As I begin my morning walk, I sense that my patience can no longer sustain my wait. The optimism in my heart is battling the pessimism in my mind. Faith and fear are having a duel; and fear is a ruthless aggressor.

I need help. I need my Lord to be at hand. I need Him to come. Suddenly, I realize He has heard the cry of my heart. He is whispering, "Be patient," by opening my spiritual eyes to the lessons of patience surrounding me.

As far as I can see—to the north, south, east, and west—are fields and farmers. Once the fields are planted, farmers are forced to be patient. At the mercy of weather, economics, and other threats, they can only do that which is within their control—and then they must wait.

Looking up into the treetops, I spot an abandoned bird's nest. During the spring, I had observed the building of the nest, the incubation of eggs, the nourishing of tiny bodies through open beaks, and finally the flight of fledglings to their independence. Birds, and the animal kingdom in general, are created with an instinctive patience that is necessary for their survival.

Now my roving eyes linger on the flowerbeds. How strange that, in my work with plants—sowing, cultivating, weeding—I had missed their lesson on patience. The flower bulbs had to endure an ugly, drab appearance, followed by being buried in a dark hole, and finally playing dead while waiting for the long, frigid winter to pass. Only then, in spring, were they permitted to move toward the nurturing rains and sunlight and emerge to their eventual glorious beauty.

The vegetable garden draws my attention next. The pea pods and leaf lettuce are mature now; green beans, onions, melons, and squash will need to wait several weeks, even months, to reach their prime.

Scanning the yard, apple trees appear to be dotted with green marbles. In time, the fruit on the trees will ripen and be transformed into pies, sauce, and jelly. But for now, patience and waiting are inevitable.

In the distance, I see the home of my daughter and son-in-law. They too are waiting. Anticipating the birth of their first child in the early fall, they are going to prenatal appointments, birthing sessions and parenting classes. Knowing that a premature birth would jeopardize their baby, they are willingly exercising patience.

Heading back toward our home now, I realize how refreshed I feel. My patience has been renewed, and my heart has been strengthened. The Lord is at hand and is beside me during the waiting. His bounteous patience will be sufficient for my need.

Dear Lord, Your eye is everywhere and You are always on hand to meet my need. Thank You for revealing that waiting and patience are often part of Your Divine plan. Please help strengthen my patience so that I can benefit from times of waiting. Amen.

Surgery and Follow-Up

Nurse-Teacher Heroine

Let me teach you; for I am gentle and humble, and you shall find rest for your souls.

—Matthew 11:29 (TLB)

With the date of my surgery near, my husband and I were on our way to the hospital Center for Breast Care for the presurgery class with a nurse clinician, whose role today would be to educate us in preparation for my upcoming surgery. It was an appointment we were actually looking forward to.

Settling into the passenger seat of our car, I decided to relax and savor this hour free from responsibility. It felt almost blissful to just gaze out the window and let my thoughts meander. I wondered about the nurse who would be our teacher today—this nurse-teacher who would join the succession of educators who have influenced my life.

My mother, teaching in a small rural school while my father served overseas as a World War II soldier, was the first "professional" teacher I knew. Influenced by her immigrant parents, she placed a high value on education. It was she who motivated and encouraged me to set high educational goals during my school years and beyond. Instilling in me a love for learning and a respect for educators, she became my first "teacher heroine."

I visualized those elementary and secondary teachers who most influenced me in becoming the person I am today. Upon reflection, I realized they all were passionate about their subject matter and its significance. They were effective not only in teaching their subject matter, but also in communicating their respect and caring for me as an individual. They were the few who stood out from the rest and became my teacher heroes and heroines.

Post-high school education over the years brought me more teachers, often with titles to signify doctorate degrees. The teacher who made the most significant impact on my life, however, taught me as an employer rather than as a classroom professor. Dr. Fred Smith was a biochemistry professor and researcher. During my junior year at the university, I worked part-time washing the laboratory equipment used by his graduate students.

One day while I was washing test tubes, he stopped to chat and asked, "Sharon, have you tried the great experiment?" Noticing my puzzled expression, he went on to explain the great experiment as trusting Jesus Christ to be my Savior and Lord and inviting Him to guide my life. He suggested I consider accepting God's gift of salvation and eternal life by professing my genuine belief in His son Jesus.

Although I initially rejected Dr. Smith's words, I pondered them with increasing interest over the next few weeks. I realized that although I had been baptized and confirmed and knew *about* Jesus, I didn't have a vital, personal relationship with Him. I also didn't have an inner assurance that—upon my eventual death—I would be with Him for eternity. Late one night soon after that, I recognized my longing to fill the spiritual void in my life and took the leap of faith Dr. Smith had spoken of. I knelt down, asked God to forgive my sins, told Him I believed Jesus died for my sins so that I could have eternal life, gave my life to Him, and asked Him to help me become the woman He created me to be.

My Christian faith, previously external, became internalized. Although people's journeys of faith vary, for me the sincere prayer of that night was the turning point of my life—spiritually and otherwise. Dr. Smith became my faith-teacher hero.

My reminiscing could have continued, but we were almost at our destination. With the hospital now in view, the thoughts of my many teachers over the years converged to one thought—what we would learn at the Center for Breast Care—and one teacher—the nurse clinician who would teach us.

Later in the afternoon, as we made our way back home from the hospital Center for Breast Care, I knew that our time there had been well spent. Our nurse clinician-teacher was all we had hoped for and more. She gently penetrated our casual surface veneer and helped us identify and address our concerns and anxieties. She reviewed my diagnosis and thoroughly answered the questions that we had previously been unprepared to ask about my upcoming lumpectomy.

Satisfied that we were ready to move on, she proceeded to give us an overview of what to expect on my surgery day—who would be involved, what each would be doing, and when and where each step would take place.

She gave special attention to a new technique, called sentinel lymph node biopsy. This technique, she explained, was developed to reduce the side effects of breast cancer surgery and could also provide important information about my breast cancer. The term *sentinel*, a military term referring to the soldiers who stand guard, is used because the sentinel lymph nodes are located in the frontline position of guarding the underarm axillary lymph nodes.

To help my surgeon locate the one or two sentinel lymph nodes, a radioactive tracer would be injected around the tumor in my breast on the morning of my surgery.

Once my surgery would begin, a blue dye would also be used to identify the sentinel nodes, which would be removed and immediately sent to the pathology lab for examination. If the nodes are determined to be cancer free, the cancer likely has not yet spread to the more distant nodes and no further nodes would be removed. If cancer cells are found in the sentinel lymph node(s), a varying number of remaining nodes would need to be excised.

Our clinical nurse had been a knowledgeable, articulate, patient, and caring teacher. My surgery was clearly important to her. I was important to her. My husband was important to her. For the duration of her time with us, she allowed us to feel as if we were the two most important people in her life. Our fear of the unknown was replaced by our knowledge of what to expect. A gold star for my nurse-teacher heroine!

Dear Lord Jesus, You are my Divine Healer and Divine Teacher hero. It seems as though You call some people to be part of Your healing team and call others to be teachers. Those who are called by You often follow Your ways—they are gentle and humble and provide rest for the soul. Today, I'm especially grateful for those You call to be nurse-teachers. May You bless their valued ministry. Amen.

Peace Beyond Understanding

The peace of God, which surpasses all understanding, will guard your hearts and your minds in Christ Jesus.
—Philippians 4:7 (NRSV)

It is still dark outside when our clock sounds its reveille, rousing my husband and me to a new day. This isn't just any day. Today is the day of my breast cancer surgery. Today is the day I have been anticipating with mixed feelings. Today is the day I will finally get rid of the menacing malignant tumor. Today is a day that will inevitably be unpleasant.

I allow myself a few moments to snuggle into the caress of our summer bedsheets. Yet, even as I am succumbing to the temptation to extend my luxurious rest, my mind is already racing ahead to the surgery room. The pathology report, including the lymph node status, will be known as a result of what happens in that room, and will dictate further treatment. But now it is time to stop resting and thinking—it is finally time for action!

After a quick shower, I realize that the simplicity of getting ready belies the complexity of the surgery ahead. It will certainly be an unadorned me that greets the medical staff today. Makeup and feminine extras are prohibited. No need to fuss with my hair—it will be covered with a sterile cap. I don't even need to take time for breakfast, as my fast must be strictly adhered to. I grab a small bag of reading material and personal items and head out our familiar door—into a not-so-familiar day.

Our headlights penetrate the soft darkness of the waning night as we head west toward the Twin Cities. Soon we leave the country roads and merge onto the highway. Looking over my shoulder to the east, I see the awakening dawn; it whispers, "There is no turning back now." There is no stopping this day, July 19. It is beginning as surely as the sun is rising.

I glance at my chauffeur-husband and am filled with appreciation for him. I'm grateful that he is such a skilled, conscientious driver. Lulled by my sense of security as the car purrs along in the twilight, I nod off for a brief snooze.

Wakened by the press of congested traffic and the audible protests of my empty stomach, I feel disorientated for a moment. Then I remember where we are going and why. A few butterflies find their home in the empty hollow of my belly.

I turn to study my husband's profile. His tense jawline and clenched hands on the steering wheel reveal his challenges—maneuvering through early rush-hour traffic while dealing with his own thoughts. I wonder what he is thinking—what his fears and hopes are. Perhaps we should be using this time to talk, to share what is going on within. No, I decide. For now, we each need this time alone with our thoughts and feelings—later we will share them and pray together.

We turn into the parking ramp and find an empty stall. We are now close to the site of my surgery, which will be performed in the hospital across the street from the ramp. I have seen the sunrise of this day. By sunset, my surgery will be behind me.

My husband and I hold hands. We offer a prayer of thanks—thanks for our safe arrival at the hospital, thanks for the prayer support we are so conscious of, thanks for the peace that is enfolding us. It is the peace of God, an inner calm in the midst of a storm, which surpasses all understanding. It will guard our hearts and minds through all that this day holds.

Dear God, I don't understand how You bring the sunrise and the sunset. Neither do I understand all that transpires during a surgery day. How can I understand a peace that will guard me from the sunrise to the sunset of this day? But I don't need to understand the peace You give in order to receive it and to have it guard my heart and mind in Christ Jesus. I thank You for Your gift of peace which surpasses all understanding. Amen.

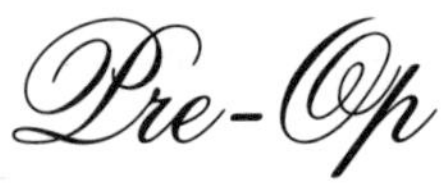

Pre-Op

Be strong and of good courage; be not frightened, neither be dismayed; for the Lord your God is with you wherever you go.

—Joshua 1:9 (RSV)

It is 9:30 A.M. and so much has already transpired that I'm having difficulty believing that my surgery day has barely reached mid-morning.

After my husband and I arrived at the hospital Breast Center at 7:00 this morning, I was summoned almost immediately to begin the day's course of action.

The ultrasound-guided procedure that placed the needle and wire in my tumor went very well. Mammograms confirmed the correct location of the wire in my breast. The radiologist sounded very pleased as he announced, "Perfect, even if I do say so myself. The wire is at the exact center of the tumor."

The relatively new sentinel-node biopsy would be part of my surgery regimen. A radioactive dye was injected into my breast and was already beginning its intended mission: seeping through the lymph ducts in my breast toward the first one or two lymph nodes encountered—those known as sentinel lymph nodes—to distinguish them by the time the surgery would take place.

A staff person from the Surgery Center arrived to escort us here, the holding room. I wondered why it was named the *holding* room. I tried to recall the various definitions of the word *hold*. Was I being held as in "detained from escape" or held as in "kept in position and supported"? Suppressing the momentary urge to flee my captors as prompted by the former definition, I accepted the intention of the latter definition and settled into my chair.

A woman with a staff badge entered the room and identified herself as my day nurse. After taking my blood pressure and temperature, she told us, "You are on your own until ten o'clock or so when the various operating room personnel will come and introduce themselves to you." With a reassuring smile, she departed from the room.

After discussing how to use our thirty unscheduled minutes, my husband left in pursuit of a daily newspaper. Alone now with my thoughts, I reflect upon the nurse's parting words, "You are on your own." But I am not on my own at all. God has been with me all morning and is, in fact, with me at this very moment.

Soon Colin will return with the newspaper and our son Aaron will arrive—Aaron with his tall, muscular frame disguising his teddy-bear heart. He'll have a smile and a joke and will communicate in his own way, "I love you. I'll be praying. I'll be with Dad keeping vigil during your surgery." The operating room personnel will come too. They will introduce themselves and acquaint us with their roles in the surgery procedure.

Eventually, however, it will be just me being wheeled into the surgery room. I will be the one receiving anesthesia. The surgeons and assisting staff will be hovering over my body—making incisions, removing a tumor and the one or more lymph nodes. I will be the only one recovering in the recovery room.

I will be a lone woman accompanied by the omnipresent God—the God whose presence I am aware of within and around. He is helping me be strong and courageous. I need not be frightened nor dismayed, for the God who brought me safely to the hospital and stayed with me at the Breast Center and the Surgery Center holding room will also be with me during surgery and recovery. My God is with me wherever I go and I am never truly alone.

Dear God, You are the Great Physician who is omnipresent and omnipotent. I receive Your gifts of inner peace, strength, and good courage. I accept Your promise to be with me wherever I go. I place my trust in You. Amen.

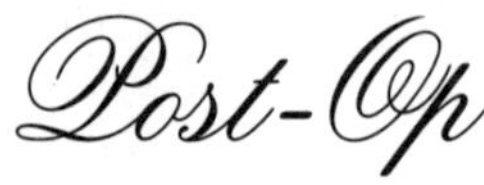

Post-Op

The Lord will sustain him upon his sickbed; in his illness, Thou dost restore him to health.

—Psalm 41:3

My eyelids fluttered open for a moment—just long enough to note my son Aaron's anxious expression—and then they were seduced back into compliance with anesthetic-induced sleep.

Another brief awakening followed. I heard a nurse urging my husband to go home and return in the morning. My husband came near me, trying to tell me that all went well, that he'd see me in the morning . . . maybe more. I drifted off again into my dizzy slumber.

I roused again, but everything was amiss. My senses were all awry. I felt light-headed and nauseated. I felt the urge to urinate, but I couldn't move. I had no comprehension of time. I was hooked up to something. Two other somethings were on my legs—progressively compressing and then releasing, over and over again. I was disorientated and definitely out of my comfort zone.

* * *

Now I am awakening to improved perceptions and am relieved to see a nurse entering my room. I groggily tell her about my nausea and need to use the bathroom. She is compassionate and responsive as she assists me to the bathroom and back. After answering my most pressing questions—the somethings on my legs are to prevent blood clots and the time is 11:30 P.M.—she arranges the bedding around me and leaves.

I realize it's been a long time since the sun rose on my surgery day. The sun has now set. It hasn't been the most pleasant day; but the surgery is over and tomorrow the sun will rise on a new day—the beginning of being restored to health. For now, I only want to sink again into the softness of my pillow and the depths of my sleep.

> **Dear Protector, I'm so grateful that You never sleep, but are always present and alert. Even when I am most helpless and vulnerable on my sickbed, I can trust You to sustain me and restore me to health. I need You. I thank You. Amen.**

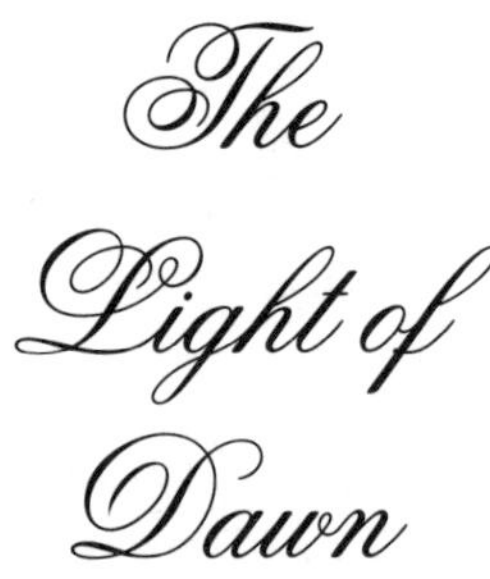

But the path of the righteous is like the light of dawn, that shines brighter and brighter until the full day.

—Proverbs 4:18

In the wee hours of the morning, I awoke—clear-headed, mildly nauseated, and needing to use the bathroom. While pressing the button to summon a nurse or assistant, I surveyed my surroundings. I had the room to myself, it was still dark outside, and the "somethings" on my legs were still compressing and releasing—preventing blood clots, I recalled.

A woman entered wearing a colorful smock and a demeanor that suggested she actually enjoyed being on duty while most people slept. She was pleasant and accommodating as she prepared me for my solo trek to the bathroom and back. "In just a few more hours, I'll be able to take these off," she assured me as she wrapped and adjusted the somethings on my legs and left the room.

Resting again, I was briefly aware of various sounds drifting into my room from the corridor and street. Although my mind was becoming restless, my body had not yet satisfied its seemingly insatiable appetite for sleep and coerced my mind to comply with its plea for yet more slumber.

* * *

I awake to the light of dawn. Hearing the sounds of dawn penetrating through the hospital wall, I recognize them as coming from the early morning traffic. They are the same sounds I heard yesterday morning as my husband drove me to the hospital.

I visualize my husband at home, alone in our bed. I hope he is sleeping well after his long day of chauffeuring, praying, supporting, keeping vigil, processing surgery information, driving home alone, returning inquiring phone calls, and tending to the needs of our dog, Mandy, and our cat, Midnight.

Soon, he'll be awake and on his way—driving here again. A surge of love and appreciation for my husband sweeps over me and warms my being. In almost thirty-three years of marriage, the number of times we've slept apart could probably be counted on our fingers and toes. Under the bandages across my chest, my heart skips a beat as I anticipate his walking through my hospital room door.

Needing to remain on my back, I turn my head to the right and stretch my neck so I can see out the window. Yes, there is a bit more sunlight now. Time seems to pass in slow motion as I rest on my bed and absorb the sounds that are accompanying this new day dawning before my eyes. The traffic is becoming more congested now, gauged by the sounds of acceleration as the light turns green. The hospital corridor is noisier too, but I am unable to discern the origins of the sounds I hear.

As their shift draws to its final hour, those who have been working throughout the night are probably also watching the dawn of this new day. I imagine them scurrying about completing their duties before their replacements arrive. They must be eager to make their way home to their own well-deserved turn to sleep. "Thank You for this night staff," I pray silently, "and help them return home safely." "Help us return home safely too," I add, realizing that in a few hours I also will be leaving.

The sun is shining brighter now. The new day is here.

Dear God, on this morning following my surgery, I thank You for Your gift of allowing me to witness the light of dawn shining brighter and brighter until the day has arrived in its fullness. It has been a grand way to usher in this first day of the rest of my life. I bask in the warmth of Your creation and love as I begin my way to recovery. Amen.

Exhausted, Feeble, and Anxious

Encourage the exhausted, and strengthen the feeble. Say to those with anxious heart, "Take courage, fear not."

—Isaiah 35:3,4

The tranquil mood that settled over me as I arose with the sun has been disrupted by the rumbling within my stomach. I realize I am famished—for food, yes, but also for information regarding my surgery.

⁂

There is a sense of urgency within me to know the answer to one particular question: "How many lymph nodes were removed?" One or two would signify the removal of only the sentinel lymph node(s). That would mean the pathologist found no cancer cells in those crucial nodes, signaling that the remaining nodes would likely be free of cancer as well—and therefore not in need of removal. I would likely still be a Stage One cancer patient.

My mind, now fully alert, is straining to remember what my surgeon told me before surgery. He had ventured the strong probability that, based on the mammogram images, my tumor would likely be one centimeter or less. He thought we could hope for no lymph-node involvement.

Lifting the blanket and sheet covering my chest, I scrutinize my right breast and underarm region. It looks like the sore and bandaged area is larger than would be necessary for the removal of just one or two lymph nodes. I sense an anxious chill penetrating me as I lower the bedclothes.

"Soon there will be a shift change," I whisper to myself as my need to know the answer to my question begins to consume me. I strategize, "My night nurse has been so kind and accommodating; perhaps she will be willing to reveal my lymph-node status." I buzz for her and wait. And wait. And wait. She appears at my door, as smiling and cordial as before. "I'm wondering if my chart indicates how many lymph nodes were removed?" I inquire in a calm, steady voice that belies the frantic pounding of my heart.

She is studying my chart now, as I simultaneously study her face for clues. With an expressionless face, she responds, "It says that eleven lymph nodes were removed." Nodding to communicate her pleasure in being able to oblige once more, she smiles and leaves.

I feel nauseated as I rest my head on the pillow and try to process her reply. Her answer was relayed so free of emotion, in so matter-of-fact a manner—she must not know the significance of the number she has just revealed. She must not be aware that her kind gesture has brought worrisome news. She must not realize that the mere number she just uttered will make a major impact on my future. She must not fathom that by heeding my request she has crushed my Pollyanna optimism. She must not know that, in likelihood, her response has communicated, "You are now a *Stage Two* cancer patient."

I am numb with concern. I feel confused, uncertain what my further treatment will entail. How many of the lymph nodes removed will reveal cancer? One? All? What about my pathology report? Will that be disappointing too? How long will I have to wait before getting the answers I want—or don't want—to hear? Suddenly, I realize that my questions are draining my strength.

As I make my way to the bathroom and back, I'm dismayed by my weakness. I settle my feeble body into the bed once more. The breakfast tray is delivered—an unusual assortment of liquids and easy-to-digest foods. My earlier ravishing hunger is now dulled by anxiety.

Exhausted, feeble, anxious. That is my condition now. I'm grateful for the prayers being offered on my behalf today. I'm grateful for the privacy of this room. I'm grateful for this time to adjust and respond to my state of being before my husband arrives. I need to be alone with God for awhile. I need to look to God for the strength, courage, and peace of mind I'll need to continue my journey toward restored health.

Dear God, You are my source of encouragement when I'm exhausted—physically, emotionally and spiritually. You are able to strengthen me when I am feeble. You know my anxious heart and You tell me, "Take courage and fear not." Though uncertain of my pathology report and future course of treatment, I continue to place my trust and hope in You. Amen.

Preparations for Discharge

"The Lord himself goes before you and will be with you; he will never leave you or forsake you. Do not be afraid; do not be discouraged."

—Deuteronomy 31:8

Preparations are being made for me to be discharged. I am given my clothing and the small bag of personal supplies from home I was advised to bring "just in case you're kept overnight." As the nurse motions toward the bathroom, she hands me a package of warmed personal cleansing cloths.

"You can use these for sponge-bathing. You'll find them soothing and refreshing. We'll be sending a supply with you to use your first several days at home too," she says.

Alone in the bathroom, I remove my hospital gown and study the woman reflected in the mirror. She bears little resemblance to the woman who crossed the street from the parking lot to the hospital barely twenty-four hours ago. Her hair is askew and matted, her face pale, and the right side of her chest and underarm area are dressed with gauze and tape. And what is that long tube protruding from the breast area and ending with a bulb-like receptacle taped to her side?

Resigned to the reality that the woman in the mirror is indeed me, and that I certainly won't be mistaken for a beauty queen as I exit the hospital, I begin to prepare for my discharge. I savor the luxury of freshly brushed teeth, despite the nagging awareness of discomfort as I move my right arm through the familiar motions.

I suspiciously eye the bulky warm package given me by the nurse and cautiously remove the contents—thick, hot, fresh-scented cloth-like paper cleansers. As I glide the cloths over my stale skin, they freshen and revive my spirit as well as my body.

My attempt to style my hair proves futile; but a touch of lipstick helps me look a bit more presentable. Recalling the nurse's directive, "no bra today," I'm grateful to be spared the painful maneuver of putting it on. Glad that I was advised during my pre-surgery orientation to wear loose, comfortable pants and a buttoned, rather than pullover shirt, I dress in the same clothes I wore briefly yesterday. I successfully meet the challenge of putting on my socks and shoes. Looking in the mirror, I can't help but smile at the pathetic-looking "after" image I'm forced to settle for in my makeover attempt.

The nurse begins my aftercare instructions just as my husband walks into the room. His affectionate greeting tells me that he is happy to see me in spite of my frumpy appearance. After being introduced to Colin, the nurse directs her attention to both of us as she carefully teaches me how to empty the fluid receptacle, measure and record its contents, clean and reattach it "twice every day." Next she demonstrates how to cleanse the area where the drainage tube has been inserted into my body and gives me bathing instructions: "You won't be able to shower until your first follow-up appointment with your surgeon. Just sponge bathe with the disposable cleansers we provided or tub bathe in a few inches of water."

Finally, all of the various instructions are finished and the discharge papers are signed. Colin is asked to bring our car to the front of the hospital and I am given a wheelchair ride to meet him. My morning nurse helps me into our car and sends us on our way with her cheery farewell. I am now a *discharged* breast cancer surgery patient!

> **Dear Lord, even as I've prepared for discharge, You've been with me, for You never leave or forsake me. Now as I go home to heal from the surgery, You are going before me. I do not need to be afraid or discouraged. I'm so grateful for Your all encompassing love and care. Amen.**

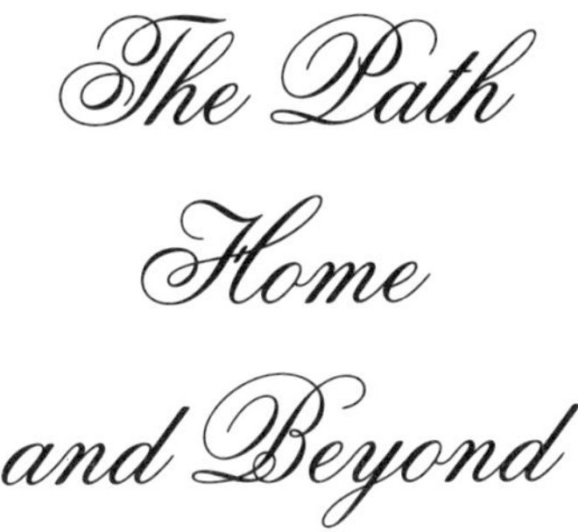

The Path Home and Beyond

In all thy ways acknowledge him and he shall direct thy paths.
—Proverbs 3:6 (KJV)

Relieved to be homeward-bound following my discharge from the hospital, I nestle into the car seat and against the headrest. I tilt my head, first to enjoy conversation with my husband, then to look out my window and watch the city sights.

After dozing for awhile, I awaken to the realization that we are now out of the city and on the familiar highway that leads to home. Cars are whizzing by, carrying people on their way somewhere for something. Farmers are busy going about their fieldwork. All are oblivious to us, to our reason for being on the highway today, to my returning home to recover from breast cancer surgery. Somehow the corn in the fields seems so much taller than it did yesterday morning. Was it just yesterday morning that we drove by these same fields?

I wonder how many times I have traveled this highway, these country roads—this well-known path that culminates at our driveway. Hundreds? Thousands? Yet, in an eerie sort of way, this morning feels like the first time.

Soon we will drive into our yard and will be greeted by our faithful welcoming committee of two. Mandy, our German shepherd dog, will uncurl from her favorite position on the patio and wag her tail as she comes to be acknowledged. Our aging tomcat, Midnight, following suit, will stretch and yawn as he sacrifices his snooze in the morning sun to meander over and meow his hope of being stroked.

We'll all walk the worn path leading from our parking spot under the shade of the gnarled old tree to our home's entrance. We'll be our usual single file parade—Mandy will lead the way, I'll follow, Colin will be just behind me carrying my overnight bag, and Midnight will bring up the rear. We could walk the route blindfolded.

Yesterday I walked the path to surgery. This morning the surgery is over, the tumor is gone, eleven lymph nodes have been removed, and I'm walking the path to home and recovery. There are many paths to walk in life—some old and familiar, others new and uncertain. I thank God for the old and familiar paths that sometimes in the past have seemed mundane and bothersome, but today offer comfort and intimacy.

And the new and uncertain path before me now? I acknowledge God in all my ways and ask Him to direct this and all of my future paths.

Dear God, I thank You for the blessing of my old and familiar paths. As new, uncertain paths loom before me, I acknowledge You as my Lord and Divine Navigator. I ask You to direct my paths as I choose to follow You. Amen.

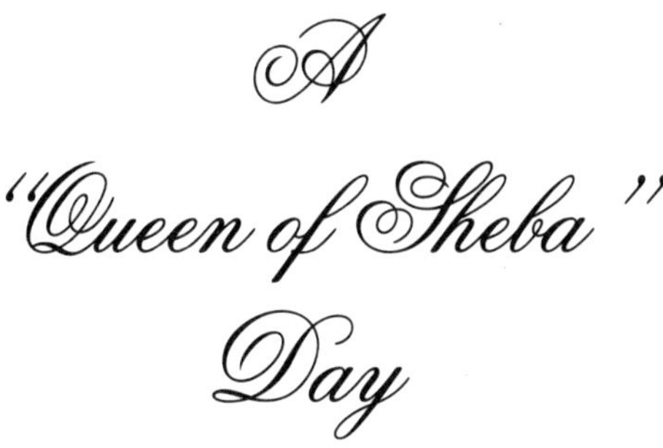

A "Queen of Sheba" Day

This is the day which the Lord has made; let us rejoice and be glad in it.
—Psalm 118:24

It has been a "Queen of Sheba" day, this first day of recovery at home. I chuckle to myself as I recall the history of my Queen of Sheba days. Often an obstinate daughter during my early teen years, I especially clashed with my mother on Saturdays. Saturday was the primary workday in our family and there always seemed to be a long list of tasks to be accomplished before my siblings and I could relax. Mom was an early riser, whose energy peaked in the morning and waned later in the day. Her plan was to begin the workday early to ensure the completion of all tasks.

I, on the other hand, viewed Saturday morning as my opportunity to sleep later than usual. My plan was to begin my tasks whenever I chose to get up. I'd linger in bed with my daydreams and procrastinate until, finally, my mother would yell up the stairs, "Who do you think you are, the Queen of Sheba? Get up *now!* There's lots of work to be done today!"

After my marriage, I happened to relate the Saturday morning saga to my husband. He urged me to take occasional days off from my responsibilities to spend as I chose. These therapeutic, luxurious days were dubbed my Queen of Sheba days.

Having been told during my presurgery orientation to rest the day after my surgery, I'd decided to make my postsurgery day a Queen of Sheba recovery day. Our master bedroom is in a preremodeling state, but our daughter's former room now is maintained as a lovely guestroom. With its antique furnishings and many windows, it would indeed be a room that would allow me to feel like a queen.

* * *

Entering the room this morning, I was welcomed by its sunny, cheerful ambiance—complete with my husband's thoughtful surprise of pink-blossomed azalea plants and roses. As I settled into the sheets, the discomfort and fatigue of my body was soon overshadowed by my sense of being loved and pampered.

The afternoon was filled with rest and reassuring care. When my husband brought up the mail, I savored each card addressed to me. The images on the cards were beautiful or humorous and the words served as a healing balm. Each promise of further prayers for my recovery nourished my spirit. I felt like I was floating, content and serene, on the prayers of those who cared about me.

The occasional ringing of the telephone brought inquiries about my well-being, messages of encouragement, and more assurances of prayer. "Soft foods, nothing too spicy," I heard my husband responding to whoever made the late afternoon call. Grinning, he came to my door to tell me his news: "That was Matt calling from work. He wants to get groceries and make supper for us tonight. It should be interesting!"

I basked in the joy of Matt's unsolicited offer to be our chef for the evening. I tried to visualize our son, recently back from Army Reserve deployment and living with us for the summer before beginning college in the fall. I imagined him leaving his work site, tired and soiled, and heading to the grocery store. I wondered what he would choose and how he would prepare it. As my husband had commented, "It should be interesting!"

Once home, Matt insisted that his dad and I relax together in the living room and watch television while he clanged and banged and opened and shut doors in the kitchen. With tantalizing aromas preceding our escort to the table, Matt proudly served his meal—pork chops with green beans and carrots for Colin and himself; rice with chicken, Jell-O cup, and a bowl of pineapple pieces topped with a raspberry for me. It was a feast fit for a queen—the Queen of Sheba.

Though a day of soreness and fatigue, this first day of recovery has also been an extraordinary day in another way. I have felt pampered, cared for, and loved. I have felt like royalty! This day I have been lavishly reminded that I *am* royalty—I am a daughter of The King!

Dear God, You are the King of Kings and Lord of Lords. Thank You for making this day so memorable by reminding me in so many ways that I am Your treasured daughter. Thank You for the dear ones who were Your channels of love. I am filled with rejoicing and gladness. Amen.

Pathology Report

"And which of you being anxious can add a single cubit to his life's span? Therefore do not be anxious for tomorrow; for tomorrow will care for itself. Each day has enough troubles of its own."

—Matthew 6:27,34

July 27 is here. It's been eight days since my surgery—eight days of healing while waiting for today's significant appointments. By mid-afternoon my husband and I will be informed of the facts contained in my pathology report—the prognosis that will steer the course of my tomorrows.

Because my initial appointment with the oncologist is set for 10 A.M. and the follow-up appointment with my surgeon isn't until 1:40 P.M., Colin and I decide to have a leisurely luncheon date during the interim. We are optimistic and have high hopes for the news the day will bring.

⁂

It's been a good news, bad news, see-saw kind of day. The oncologist began the appointment with an upbeat tone as he shared the apparent good news that the report indicated a 1 by 0.8 by 0.7 centimeter tumor, the size of a small pea—a Stage One size. Colin and I exchanged quick glances of relief. We were hoping I would be a Stage One cancer patient.

The oncologist went on to explain that only one of the eleven lymph nodes removed—one of the two sentinel lymph nodes to be exact—was cancerous. Yes, it was good news that only one lymph node was involved. It was also good news that the size of the metastatic focus in the one node was very small—one millimeter, the size of a pen point.

The subtle change in the oncologist's demeanor cued me to a shift in the topic of the news: The reality of the one malignant node plus other significant factors in the report had moved me from a Stage One to a Stage Two cancer patient. My husband's furrowed brow bespoke his intensified concern. My heart sank and pulled my high hopes with it. Once again my ability to concentrate was being challenged by a cacophony of emotions.

Had the pathology report been in a foreign language, it would have been almost as comprehensible. I understood only a few of the words as I strained my ears trying to absorb what we were being told. I began to take notes, but the oncologist kindly prodded me just to listen—he would gladly write as he spoke.

I had not just one, but two kinds of cancer cells—intraductal and invasive. After explaining the difference, the oncologist shifted his focus to the topic of recurrence. The dreaded word *metastasis*, defined as the spread of cancer from one part of the body to another, was illustrated as he drew arrows on his notepad from the word breast to the words lung, bones, and liver. These were the incurable cancers, he noted.

The oncologist went on to inform us of the five predictors of metastastic spread:

1. Age of patient—Good news! The prognosis is better for postmenopausal women. At the age of fifty-seven, I am postmenopausal.
2. Size of tumor—Good news! The one centimeter size of my tumor was in my favor.
3. Lymph-node status—Good news and bad news. The good news was that only one node was positive for cancer. The bad news was that even one positive lymph node signals caution.

4. Estrogen receptor status—Bad news. My cancerous cells were estrogen-receptive negative, meaning that I would not be a candidate for hormonal therapy. The majority of women with breast cancer have cancerous cells that are estrogen-receptive positive. They are eligible to be treated with estrogen blocking drugs such as tamoxifen.
5. Growth rate of the cancer cells—Bad news. On the Nottingham scale of one to three, one being the slowest growing and three being the fastest growing, my cells were a three.

Statistics showed that, with the prescribed treatment of surgery, chemotherapy, and radiation, I would have a 20 percent chance of recurrence within five years. I summed up the data to conclude that I am a Stage Two cancer patient with the possibility of aggressive, stray cancer cells that can't be blocked by hormone therapy drugs and therefore could metastasize and kill me within five years.

The conscientious oncologist handed me the notes he had been taking as he talked. They were illegible to me. Perhaps I was simply too dazed to read his or anyone's handwriting. Even if I could have read his writing, could I grasp the message the words, numbers, and diagrams conveyed? Would I even want to comprehend fully what he had so carefully explained? Where was the good news? It seemed to have been overtaken by the bad.

Stunned and anxious, my husband and I somehow found our way to a restaurant. How foolish we had been, how into denial of the possibility of bad news, to have actually been looking forward to a luncheon date between appointments. While we forced down a tasteless meal, our minds were occupied with digesting something other than food—the unpalatable pathology report.

Weary and worried, we returned to the clinic for the 1:40 appointment with the surgeon. As sensitively as possible, he reviewed the pathology report and reiterated the oncologist's interpretation and recommendations.

He also delivered more news—bad news. The tumor strands were too close to the edge of the tissue removed during surgery. There would need to be a second surgery. A wider margin surrounding the tumor mass would need to be excised. Colin and I would make the final decision regarding the extent of the excision. The surgery was scheduled for August 25—almost another month to wait! We would use the time to pray and seek additional professional opinions regarding the extent of the second surgery.

We drove home too wiped out to converse. It took all of our energy to cope with the developments of the day. Feeling too exhausted to attend a scheduled supper at the home of relatives, I sent my husband on without me. I needed to rest, to recover from this day, and to summon up the strength and will to face another.

Feeling faint, I lay down. Was my weakness due to an empty, nauseated stomach? To being overwhelmed by the confusing language and foreboding conclusions of the pathology report? To the replacing of optimism with draining anxiety? From the recesses of my besieged mind, the words of Jesus recorded in Matthew 6 emerged to rescue me from the brink of despair.

Yes, this day has had its share of troubles. Yet, Jesus' words are able to sooth like a healing balm and calm my anxious worries for tomorrow. Whether my life span is five years or less, or twenty-five years or more, being anxious won't add a "single cubit" to it. Therefore, I resolve not to be anxious for tomorrow, for tomorrow will care for itself. I drift off to sleep, relinquishing my tomorrows to God's care.

Dear Lord, even on the worst, most troublesome days, You are beside me and within me to buffer and sustain and give hope for a better tomorrow. Please help me deal with my anxiety and find my way through this confusing maze of breast cancer tomorrows. I love You and need You. I place my faith in You. Amen.

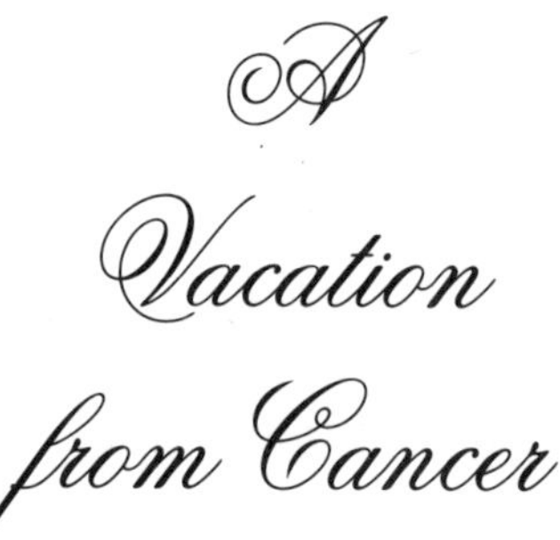

A Vacation from Cancer

For everything there is a season, and a time for every matter under heaven . . . a time to weep, and a time to laugh; a time to mourn and a time to dance.

—Ecclesiastes 3:1,4

My husband and I were finishing our lunch when the telephone rang. Colin answered the phone and responded to my inquisitive look by silently mouthing, "It's Dennis and Angela calling from Canada." My curiosity, momentarily satisfied by the knowledge that Colin's brother and sister-in-law were the *who*, peaked again as I listened to Colin's end of the conversation and tried to decipher the *why*.

Finally, Colin concluded the long distance exchange with, "I'll talk it over with Sharon and get back to you."

"Well?" I eventually probed, a tad chagrined by Colin's prolonged silence. He obviously was pondering the call and considering how to best share it with me.

Deciding on the straightforward approach, he began. "Dennis and Angela called while driving across Canada on a business trip. They're planning to take a few days of R and R at a resort in northern Minnesota when they get back. They want to know if we'd like to join them. What do you think?"

My thoughts began to bounce like a beach ball set in motion. Rest and recuperation—we surely could use some of that! I had previously been to the resort favored by Dennis and Angela, and I could visualize the picturesque setting, varied recreation options, and exceptional meals it offered.

But, looking down at the drainage tube that was protruding from my chest, I thought, "This invitation couldn't have come at a worse time. I'm still struggling with soreness and fatigue, reeling from my disappointing pathology report, and dealing with this bothersome drainage tube."

The ball in my mind bounced back and forth as I pondered and stewed, and stewed and pondered. Finally the ball landed on a profound thought: This was not the worst time for a vacation; it was the *best* time for a vacation—a vacation from cancer!

I was at my saturation point with facts, anxieties, treatments, and everything else related to breast cancer. Three days and two nights without one word pertaining to breasts or cancer from any of us—that would be a real vacation. Perhaps if nothing was spoken or read there about cancer, I could even give my *mind* a vacation from it.

I shared my thoughts and feelings with Colin. He wholeheartedly supported my vacation plan and telephoned Dennis and Angela with the go-ahead to make reservations. Recently, I had become so accustomed to having something to dread that I'd forgotten what it felt like to have something to be excited about. "Whoopee!"

* * *

With the uncommonly perfect summer weather holding us in its embrace for yet a third day, Dennis, Angela, Colin, and I are leaving our resort haven for the homeward drive. The four of us have wined and dined, strolled and pontooned, read and napped, chatted and laughed.

As a couple, Colin and I have welcomed this vacation as an early anniversary celebration. Ignoring the tube protruding from my chest, we have honeymooned and reminisced over highlights of our almost thirty-three years of marriage.

Now, even if reluctantly, I am ready to leave my brief fantasy-land, and face the real world of continuing breast cancer treatment. I have had my time to weep and mourn, and will likely do so again. I have also found my time to laugh and dance, and will do so again, and again, and again throughout the remaining seasons of my life.

Dear Heavenly Father, You are Lord of all seasons and all times. You never take a vacation from me, but are with me always. You are the reason I can laugh and dance in the midst of tears and loss. You are my Divine dance partner—during this life and into eternity. Amen.

Second Opinion—Second Surgery

And this is the confidence which we have before Him, that, if we ask anything according to His will, He hears us. And if we know that He hears us in whatever we ask, we know that we have the requests which we have asked from Him.

—1 John 5:14-15

And your ears will hear a word behind you, "This is the way, walk in it."

—Isaiah 30:21

Now to Him who is able to do exceedingly abundantly beyond all that we ask or think, according to the power that works within us, to Him be the glory in the church and in Christ Jesus to all generations forever and forever. Amen.

—Ephesians 3:20-21

Soon after my first postoperative appointments with the oncologist and surgeon, my husband and I took a brief "vacation from cancer." It had been a grand time of rest and relaxation, but now it was back to the reality of breast cancer treatment. Looming over us was the crucial decision about a second surgery.

As the surgeon interpreted my pathology report during the postoperative appointment, he had informed us of my need to schedule a second surgery. He explained that there were cancer cells within one millimeter—only a pen-point's width from both the inferior/medial and the anterior margins of the tissue excised during my lumpectomy.

My two surgery choices were to excise a wider margin of tissue around the original surgery site—and hope for no further cancer cells—or to have a mastectomy. In his experience, the surgeon had disclosed, most of those who had opted for the less invasive surgery had needed a third surgery—the mastectomy—because of cancer cells found in the excised tissue. He also noted that a third surgery would mean a further delay in commencing the next phase of treatment.

Sensitive to our expressions of disappointment, and our hesitancy to make the decision immediately, he kindly suggested that we set the surgery date, consider our options, and inform him of our choice at my next postoperative appointment.

Burdened by the heavy weight of this new, unexpected decision, Colin and I discussed our thoughts and feelings. We were in agreement in what we *didn't* want—we didn't want a mastectomy if it wasn't necessary, and we didn't want a third surgery with a postponement of chemotherapy.

Although my surgeon suspected that there were additional cancer cells near the margin, he wasn't certain. Only God knew whether there were cancer cells present. We decided to ask God to clearly show us His will regarding our decision. After joining hands in fervent prayer, we waited in expectancy for God's guidance.

Later that day, we recalled our son Aaron having mentioned a few weeks earlier that two of his clients were breast cancer surgeons. When he had shared with them his concern for me following my diagnosis, they both had given Aaron their home telephone numbers along with the invitation for me to call if I needed their input.

I dialed the number of the first surgeon and was greeted with genuine caring. After listening to my pathology report over the telephone, he indicated that he would choose the mastectomy. He added that he preferred to err on the side of caution. He also stated that because he had moved into a management position, he was no longer performing breast surgery. After informing me that Aaron's other breast surgeon client was a nationally noted pioneer in the latest frontiers of breast cancer surgery, he recommended that I contact him before making my decision.

The following day, it occurred to Colin that his former college housemate was now practicing and teaching surgery at a university hospital in another state. That evening he reached our mutual friend by telephone and shared our situation. Our surgeon friend was eager to assist in any way possible. Upon receiving a copy of my pathology report, he along with a colleague who specialized in breast cancer surgery reviewed and discussed my data. They both leaned toward the mastectomy option. However, his colleague, the breast cancer specialist, had urged us to seek the opinion of a nationally acclaimed surgeon in Minnesota. My husband and I gasped when we heard the surgeon's name—it was the same name as Aaron's other surgeon client!

The next evening I called the home of the surgeon whom his three colleagues were referring to as a higher authority. My heart was racing with anxiety when he answered the telephone, but his warm concern immediately put me at ease and I proceeded to explain my dilemma. After asking me numerous questions pertaining to my pathology report, his response was: "In my opinion, a mastectomy would be premature based on the data in your report. I recommend excising a wider margin of tissue."

As Colin and I prayed prior to my next postoperative appointment, we both sensed a deep inner peace regarding choosing the less invasive surgery. I was quite uneasy, however, about the prospect of informing my surgeon that our choice differed from his recommendation. I asked several women from our congregation to pray that my positive relationship with the surgeon wouldn't be undermined by the decision Colin and I had made.

Prayers—both for a confirmation of our choice and for a positive response from my surgeon—were answered "abundantly, beyond all that we asked or thought." When I told my physician of our decision, based on the input of the noted breast cancer surgeon, he exclaimed in amazement, "He was my surgery teacher! We'll do what he recommends."

Oh, by the way, the second surgery was like the grand finale to God's orchestration of answered prayer. Only a local anesthesia with intravenous sedation was needed for my 8 A.M. outpatient surgery. By 10:30 A.M. I left the hospital feeling so great that it was an effort to spend the day resting as prescribed. There were no drainage tubes protruding from my breast as after my initial surgery, my body healed quickly, and I was soon able to schedule my next phase of treatment.

The pathology report results? As soon as my surgeon received the report, he called with the good news: "The pathology report indicates that the excised tissue was free of cancer cells!" He joined my husband and me in celebrating the choice we had made—the choice that God had so clearly guided us to.

Dear God, You truly are the Great Physician. Thank You for hearing our prayer and for answering by guiding us to Your way. Thank You for the surgeons You brought into my life; I ask Your blessing upon them. Please help me to remember to come with confidence before You, my Highest Authority—not only with my prayer petitions, but also with my praise. To You be the glory. Amen.

Where Did I See God in My Life Today?

"Do not fear, for I have redeemed you; I have called you by name; you are Mine! When you pass through the waters, I will be with you; and through the rivers, they will not overflow you. When you walk through the fire, you will not be scorched, nor will the flame burn you. For I am the Lord your God . . . ."

—Isaiah 43:1-3

It is another transition time: a healing time before the next phases of treatment commence. My surgeries are behind me, chemotherapy and radiation lie ahead.

I recall the day a dear friend called to chat and inquire how I was doing, how I was *really* doing. I wonder if she realized how incredible it was to be given the freedom to be totally candid and honest?

As we had wound down our conversation, Sylvia ventured a suggestion: "At the close of every day, ask yourself this question—'Where did I see God in my life today?'—and then journal your response." "Well . . . I'll try it," I had replied tentatively.

After several weeks of asking and journaling, I've been amazed that there are no blank pages. It is as though I have grown antennae that are attuned to a greater awareness of God's presence in every aspect of my life. Many days, I see Him in the nearness, the artistry, the soothing balm of His creation. On other days, I see or hear Him through people—a phone call, visit, or greeting card from a relative, friend, or acquaintance; or even an affirming smile or thoughtful gesture from a stranger. Sometimes, I sense His presence in an unexplainable inner peace or surge of joy. Often I feel His nearness through music or the words of a poem, an article, or a book.

The book in which I most often find God's presence is the Bible, especially in the hundreds of promises proclaimed within its covers. A scholar trained in the interpretation of Scripture would differentiate between those promises intended for everyone and those intended for a specific person or people group. I, however, find God to be present for me, to be blessing me, through any promise that He chooses.

⁂

Isaiah 43:1-3 is such a passage for me today. Although its promises were intended for the people of Israel, God is blessing me with this inherent comfort now. During my upcoming chemotherapy sessions, I will not be passing through waters and rivers, but rather rivers of liquid chemicals will be passing through me. Yet, God's promise, "I will be with you," is as true for me now during my chemotherapy as it was so long ago for the people of Israel.

While undergoing my thirty-five radiation treatments, I will not be walking through fire, but instead will have radiation rays moving through my body tissue. Nevertheless, I am invited to take comfort from God's promise, "You will not be scorched, nor will the flame burn you. For I am the Lord your God."

I especially recognize God's presence in verse 1: "Do not fear, for I have redeemed you; I have called you by name; you are Mine!" I envision myself in the future chemotherapy and radiation-treatment waiting rooms as yet unseen. I will be waiting for someone on the staff to come to the room and call, "Sharon Callister." I will rise from my chair and walk forward to receive my treatment.

In those future waiting rooms, there will be another presence—within my heart, within my spirit. I will hear another voice calling, "Sharon Callister, you are mine! Do not fear, for I have redeemed you."

Yes, I am in a transition time now between surgery and upcoming chemotherapy and radiation treatments. I need not fear, however, because I have seen God in my life today. Where did I see Him? In Isaiah 43:1-3. He and His promises are with me today and into all my tomorrows.

You are my Lord, my God. Thank You for revealing Yourself to me each day. I believe that You call me by name and that I am Yours, for You have redeemed me. I trust You to be with me and protect me now and in my future. I am filled with gratitude that You always keep Your promises. Amen.

Chemotherapy

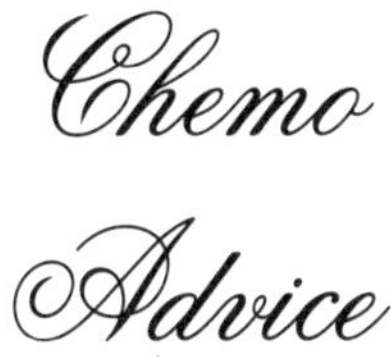

Chemo Advice

All the days of the afflicted are bad, but a cheerful heart has a continued feast.

—Proverbs 15:15

"Treat yourself to a full-body massage before each treatment. Drink lots of ginger tea before and after your treatments. Go to a movie matinee after your treatment and eat a big bag of unbuttered popcorn." The voice at the other end of the telephone bubbled over with tips to help me get through my chemotherapy treatments. Cherice, nearing the completion of her own chemotherapy, went on to explain that massage helps relax the body, making it more receptive to the treatment. Ginger is a natural antinausea spice; the movie matinee not only is something to look forward to, but also serves as a mental distraction; and popcorn bulk is believed to help reduce nausea. Before bringing our conversation to a close, she invited me to the breast cancer support group she attends: "You'll want plenty of support as you go through chemotherapy."

Another friend pulled me aside during a gathering and urged me to see a nutraceutical specialist prior to beginning chemotherapy. "You'll need to take supplements in order to keep nutrition and immunity levels up," she said.

I solicited counsel from an acquaintance who was finishing her course of treatment. "Use a day planner or journal to record your side effects, blood counts, the foods that do and don't appeal to you, and anything else that will help you maintain and plan your life during the treatments," she said; "I also recommend asking people to pray you through your treatments."

With the day of my first chemotherapy treatment quickly approaching, I carefully read the handouts and booklets I had received. There was no getting around the reality that chemotherapy would bring me physical and mental affliction. There were likely to be more bad days than good days during the course of my treatment. I glumly concluded, "Chemotherapy has come a long way, but it will likely never make the top-ten list of pleasant things to do!"

* * *

The day of my chemotherapy treatment is here. I've followed most of the advice I've received. My husband and I pray for God's protection on the road and during the procedure, and we pray for minimal side effects. We pray that God will guide the oncology staff. We thank God for those who are supporting us with their prayers and their expressions of caring. We pray for peace of mind.

The oncology nurse clinician examines the veins in my arms as she prepares for my intravenous treatment. Feeling squeamish, I look away and try to concentrate on other thoughts. I think of the prayers. I think of the facts I've learned about chemotherapy. I think of the advice I've received—and of Cherice, the first person to offer me advice. I recall her generous heart and her cheerful attitude.

I remember some of the words of advice that Charles Swindoll, a noted pastor, speaker, and author, has written on attitude: "The longer I live the more I realize the impact of attitude on life. Attitude, to me, is more important than facts. . . . The remarkable thing is we have a choice every day regarding the attitudes we will embrace for that day. . . . We cannot change the inevitable. The only thing we can do is play on the one string we have, and that is our attitude. . . . I am convinced that life is 10 percent what happens to me and 90 percent how I react to it. And so it is with you . . . we are in charge of our attitudes."

I look back at my arm now. The intravenous tube is in place. Chemicals are already traveling in my bloodstream and will move throughout my entire body. I have relinquished control of my body to God and the oncology nurse clinician. I choose to play the one string I retain control of—my attitude.

Dear God, as I begin my chemotherapy treatment, I'm grateful for the advice I have received and the people who have given it. I especially thank You for the wise advice found in Proverbs 15:15. During the bad days of my affliction, please help me to have a cheerful-hearted attitude so that I may continue to have a satisfying life. Amen.

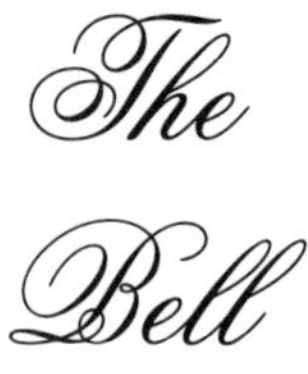

Blessed be the God and Father of our Lord Jesus Christ, the Father of mercies and God of all comfort; who comforts us in all our afflictions so that we may be able to comfort those who are in affliction with the comfort with which we ourselves are comforted by God.

—II Corinthians 1:3,4

It was the third day following my first chemotherapy treatment. My mind wanted to follow through with meeting my husband for the afterschool retirement gathering planned to honor his cousin's husband. My body, however, was wavering in its nausea, fatigue, and overall blahness. "It's mind over matter," I said aloud to press the resolution into my mind as I changed clothes and put on my wig for the first time.

No, I hadn't begun to lose my hair yet; but my unpermed, uncut hair with the wide band of grey between the bottle brown and scalp shouted that the wig would definitely be an improvement.

Greg, a co-worker of the guest of honor, was one of the first people I saw as I arrived. Greg, whose wife Mary had once been my colleague and friend. Mary's breast cancer diagnosis came late, but her Irish sense of humor and spunk, along with the support of Greg and their boys, relatives, and countless friends, carried her through a valiant race against time. Finally overcome, she had died nine months ago.

As Greg approached, I was wondering if he knew of my diagnosis. "See me before you leave; I have something for you," he said, as he went on to mingle with the other staff.

Following the party, Greg caught us in the corridor by the custodian's office. His eyes were deep with emotion as he handed me a small, unwrapped lavender box. "Someone gave this to Mary. I want you to have it now," he explained softly.

The opened box revealed an exquisite necklace—a silver-crafted bell on a delicate chain. "To honor Pauline Vinyon," the message inside the box informed me; "The Pauline's Bell necklace symbolizes awareness, hope, courage and support."

With trembling hands I held the precious bell. With quivering voice I tried to express how much the bell meant to me, how beautiful I thought it was. "I'd put it on now," I ventured, "but I'm afraid I'll catch it on my wig." Through tear-brimmed eyes that revealed his pain and belied his rugged demeanor, Greg replied, "I understand." And he did.

There weren't words adequate to describe his gift; there weren't words adequate to express my gratefulness—only the language of the eyes and a hug. The comfort of awareness, hope, courage, and support that a friend had given to Mary through Pauline's Bell were now being passed on to me as I became the next link on this sisterhood chain.

> **Dear Lord, how can I thank those who have suffered pain and loss and yet from their woundedness reach out to comfort and encourage me? Please help me to receive their gifts with grace and to trust You to bless them in ways that are beyond my capabilities. In Your perfect time and way, guide me in bringing comfort and encouragement to the next link on the chain. Amen.**

Hairs and Sparrows

Indeed, the very hairs of your head are all numbered. Do not fear; you are of more value than many sparrows.

—Luke 12:7

For some women, their hair really is their "crowning glory." As for me, I'd always thought of my hair as a hassle. Since I'd never had the knack of styling my hair, it had been an ongoing labor and expense to keep it trimmed, permed, colored, and styled. Now was honestly the first time I'd pondered what my hair meant to me. "You'll start to lose your hair two weeks after your first chemotherapy treatment," I'd been told by my oncology nurse clinician.

Fumbling through my bulging folder of breast cancer information, I found the sheets on dealing with hair loss, wigs, hats, and turbans. Advice from hair stylists and friends varied. Some said, "Take control and shave it all off yourself beforehand." Others advised, "Keep what you can for as long as you can."

As the dreaded less-hair, no-hair days drew closer, I borrowed my son-in-law's barber kit and set the date that I would "take control." As I stood looking in the mirror at my now overgrown, unpermed hair with obvious gray roots, I crumbled. I just couldn't bring myself to turn the shaver on. Over the next few days, the words, "the very hairs of your head are all numbered," kept floating through my mind, often followed by the question, "What if the number of hairs on my head is zero?"

Finally, I looked up Luke 12:7 and was startled to read the second half of the verse: "Do not fear, you are of more value than many sparrows." The point of Luke 12:7 is not how many hairs we have or don't have, but our unconditional value to God no matter what our physical condition might be.

During the next few days, I was alarmed to see brushfuls of hair, webs of wet hair on the shower stall, and clumps of hair on my pillow and clothing. I was caught in the balance between getting rid of this molting nuisance and cherishing what remained.

Then came the breezy autumn day when I rested outside on the hammock. As I ran my fingers through my hair, handfulls of hair surrendered at my touch and were caught by the wind. I imagined the delight of robins and other birds as they discovered the soft brown and gray hair tufts next spring and used them in building their nests. With purpose in my sacrifice, I shaved my remaining hair into a newspaper and spread the offering throughout our tree grove.

My God who values me more than many sparrows replaced my fear and dread with a unique and satisfying blessing.

O God, You are the creator of many hairs and many sparrows, all of which are individually numbered and valued by You. Thank You for caring about me and my hair and providing a way for me to peacefully release my hair to You. Amen.

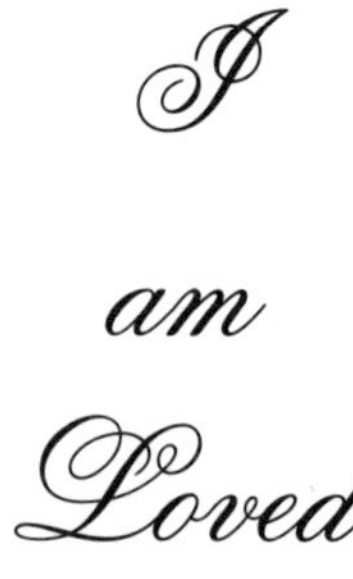

I am Loved

But now abide faith, hope, love, these three; but the greatest of these is love.
—I Corinthians 13:13

Three days following my second chemotherapy treatment, I had developed all the symptoms of a typical cold. "Rest," my body begged, but my mind was seduced to heed the call of my long-standing motto, "Mind over matter."

I had agreed to host a shower at my home and would honor my commitment "even if it kills me"—another motto I clung to as I repeatedly pushed myself beyond the boundary of fatigue.

Now I felt like I really was dying. Though my illness was not actually grave, I did end up calling the twenty-four-hour oncology help-line. Soon after the call, my husband brought me to Urgent Care, and the physician on duty informed me that I had a bacterial infection in my bronchial tubes. Fast-acting antibiotics and bed rest were his kind but firm orders.

After several days of medication, I still felt desperately ill. I loathed myself as I peppered my mind with punishing self-talk: "Why did you allow yourself to end up in this situation? When will you start listening to what your body is trying to tell you? What if this throws off your chemotherapy treatment schedule?"

Miserable, gross, ugly, unlovable, repulsive. These were the words that muddled my sluggish mind as I lay ill on my bed. Rising to use the bathroom, I wondered if I would ever feel well again. Washing my hands, I glanced in the mirror and was startled to come face to face with my image—so gaunt, so haggard, so grotesque.

As I slid back under the blankets, the bedstand clock announced that my husband would be home from work in minutes. I tried to put myself in his place—a typical stressful day at school followed by the challenge of negotiating heavy traffic, and then returning home to a wife undergoing not only chemotherapy but now also the complications of a bronchial infection.

* * *

What will he see as he enters our bedroom? A wife who is bald, chest-scarred, red-nosed, emitting chemo-tainted sweat and coughing up too-gross-to-describe mucus. In summary, a minus-a-million-sex-appeal wife!

Hearing the garage door open, I realize how embarrassed I am to have my husband—my lover—see me like this. My senses stretch to recognize the predictable sounds of Colin's return. He's taking off his shoes, then hanging his jacket in the closet. Now he is setting his lunch bag on the kitchen counter as he strides to our bedroom.

Turning my face toward the door to greet him, I am prepared for an expression of repulsion. Our eyes meet and in that moment the lying dragons in my mind are conquered by the truth in my husband's eyes: he sees only the woman he loves.

And what do I see? I see the enlightened reality that I am a woman loved—loved for who I am at the very core of my being. My husband has given me the gift of his unconditional love, the voluntary vow to love me in sickness as well as in health. He has given me a holy moment during which I begin to grasp the truth of God's boundless love for me. I am loved.

Dear God, You could have given me a glimpse of Your extraordinary love for me when I looked my most beautiful, was awarded my greatest honor, or achieved my highest goal. Instead You gave me this gift when I was most unattractive, most unremarkable, most unproductive. Thank you, my Creator, for loving me simply for who I am—Your beloved child. Amen.

Indulgences

This is the day which the Lord has made; Let us rejoice and be glad in it.
—Psalm 118:24

The simple little pleasures in life can make a great difference in one's day. Even the most mundane or bothersome day can be transformed into a time of rejoicing and gladness. A unique treat, a touch of beauty—a personal indulgence, if you will—is capable of bringing delight to a dreary day, a weary soul.

A few years ago, I began the rather odd habit of bringing home an especially pretty or interesting napkin from social gatherings I attended. I also was drawn to beautiful, unusual napkins in gift shops and boutiques. As time passed, I'd collected a cache of paper napkins in the corner of a drawer.

Now, on days when I feel a bit bland, ill, or ragged around the edges, I thumb through the napkins and select the one that conveys the emotional state I'd like to have. I add it to my beverage tray or place setting, not to actually use, but rather to replicate its mood. I'm amazed at the ability of such a simple gesture to perk up my day.

A fresh flower, bouquet, or flowering plant also carries the possibility of nurturing and brightening my inner being and outlook. Objects of visual beauty, comforting textures, poetry, Scripture, and faith-building stories too seem to possess the capacity to add charisma and lightness to my mood.

After a friend sent me a particularly uplifting compact disc, I recognized more clearly the power of music to set the tone for the day or alter the emotional climate of the hour. I treated myself to the purchase of two new CDs to enjoy while at home.

Eventually, I recognized that all of these personal indulgences were gifts of God's grace to enable me to thrive during my course of treatment. He, who knows me so completely and uniquely, is aware of each of my inner yearnings and is eager to guide towards healthy fulfillment.

Whereas my pre-breast cancer self would have tended to squelch self-indulgence, now I see that to do so would be to reject God's special treats meant just for me. I take delight in selecting a flower or plant from the supermarket or florist. I've purchased an attractive scrapbook in which to place lovely images and inspiring words. My favorite CDs are grouped together for a long-play day of audio indulgence.

A personal extravaganza might take the form of a new item of clothing or jewelry, cartoons or jokes, an engaging magazine or book, an uplifting video or movie, an art object, soothing body lotions, a learning experience, counseling, or whatever meets the need to feel feminine, nurtured, fun, interesting. This is a time in life to bask in little indulgences and enjoy them as gifts from a loving Father.

Father God, help me to not be so consumed by my breast cancer experience that I ignore my quiet inner yearnings. You know me completely and long to cheer me along my way. Help me to recognize my yearnings and the means available to satisfy them. Thank You for caring about every detail of my life and delighting in providing those perks that are especially for me. Amen.

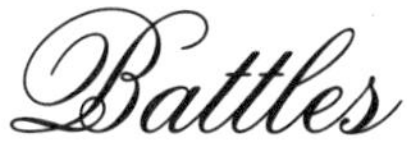

Battles

For the battle is the Lord's.
—1 Samuel 17:47

My husband was the first to notice the drama unfolding in the woods beyond our windows to the south of the townhouse we were living in during his school term. Although miniaturized by urban sprawl, this pocket of acres between housing developments held a surprising variety of trees and vegetation, birds, and other wildlife. Peering out our sunroom windows one day, we were captivated by an impromptu competition of prowess and strength within close view; we felt as if we were in the box-seat section of an arena.

During the night a large buck had ventured into the little woods and determined to claim it as his own. With the territorial instincts of generations of deer preceding him, he rubbed the tree branches with his antlers, leaving his scent of dominion. The motivation for this early morning fervor soon became apparent as a less mature buck, prepared to challenge the stag for the prize of this tiny wooded territory, strode down the hiking trail between houses.

Advance and retreat was the name of the game, as the smaller buck would advance toward the woods edge only to be bullied into retreat by the dominant male. At last the defeated younger buck acknowledged submission and retreated for the final time into the maze of homes. The victor stood guard for a few moments, then meandered out of sight into his acquired kingdom.

Today as I gaze out the same window, I realize there is no lingering evidence that a battle was staged during those brief moments of history. Several days have passed and we haven't seen any sign of either deer. The territory that seemed to be such a crucial battle trophy at the time has already been abandoned.

A parallel came to light as I realize I am gradually becoming more discriminating in my own "battles." I simply don't have the physical, emotional, or spiritual energy to continue to claim all that I think should be mine or to chase away all that I perceive to be a threat. Whether related to my health situation, my evolving personal relationships, my work, or my faith walk, I just can't take on as many battles as before.

My breast cancer experience is changing my outlook on life—many of the things that had once seemed so crucial to me are no longer important. As my course of treatment progresses, my priorities are being altered. I need this time away from the battles of my pre-breast cancer activities to contemplate my life and the direction of my future.

Like the deer, I can follow my instincts and waste precious time and energy on what isn't important or lasting, or I can turn my life and its battles over to the Lord and trust His leading.

Dear Lord, please show me those battles that are not worth fighting and help me release them to You. Guide me in discerning the battles that are worth fighting and grant me Your wisdom and strength as I fight. Help me to identify the battles that only You can fight and enlarge my faith as I trust You to be the victor. I thank and praise You, Almighty God. Amen.

Thanksgiving Feast

"Teacher, which is the great commandment of the Lord?" And He said to him, "You shall love the Lord your God with all your heart, and with all your soul, and with all your mind. This is the great and foremost commandment. The second is like it. You shall love your neighbor as yourself. On these two commandments depend the whole Law and the Prophets."

***—Matthew* 22:36-40**

Thanksgiving was approaching along with the realization that chemotherapy definitely was taking an early toll on my stamina. Checking the calendar, I counted the days between my third chemo treatment and Thanksgiving Day. Sure enough, the holiday would fall during the window of near isolation when my low white blood cell count would be at its lowest. "This will be a good year to have our kids spend Thanksgiving with their spouses' or girlfriends' families," my husband and I concluded. Just Matt, our youngest, unattached son in college, would be with us.

What a drastic change from the many years when it had been our turn to host the Thanksgiving dinner for our large extended families and to accommodate the hustle and bustle of as many as sixty people in our house. "Well, it will be different this year," I sighed, with resignation and a tinge of melancholy.

I also realized that whether cooking for sixty or for three, the traditional menu would remain the same and there would be no relatives bringing salads, pies, and other side dishes. Nope, TV turkey dinners and deli trimmings would be too drastic a change. Somehow, I would muster up the energy. God had a better plan, however . . . .

The ringing of the telephone summoned me to the almost daily check-in with Pam, my neighbor who was home recovering from her own health crisis. Her sons would be home for Thanksgiving. Her mother would be flying in to join them for the holiday. They would have tons of food, more than the five of them could possibly eat themselves. As Pam bubbled over in the exuberance of her offer, it became clear that "no" was not to be an acceptable option. It was settled. Pam's family would be preparing and delivering our Thanksgiving meal.

Thanksgiving Day arrived along with Matt, and the table was set for three. The phone call came from Pam alerting us that her sons were on the way over with our meal. The doorbell rang and the door was opened, all according to plan. But why the tears that caught me off-guard, adding an unexpected dimension to the plan? As I tried to choke back the emotions that were catching me unaware, I observed the scene in the doorway: two handsome young men, eyes sparkling with vigor and goodwill, grinning from ear to ear, laden with casseroles and aluminum foil-wrapped packages ready for the giving.

I will never forget Thanksgiving 2000. It was the year our neighbors lived out the Great Commandment and transformed our holiday meal into a feast of thanks giving.

God of all, thank You for Your commandment to love our neighbors as ourselves so that givers and recipients can be blessed with the abundant joy and thanksgiving that comes with being part of Your Divine Plan. Amen.

The Race I Didn't Plan to Enter

Let us run with patience the race that is set before us, looking unto Jesus the author and finisher of our faith.
—Hebrews 12:1,2 (KJV)

After nine weeks of chemotherapy, I can't face another day of looking at my bald head, of eating flavorless meals caused by chemo-damaged taste buds. I'm sick of feeling sick. Instead of running with patience the race set before me, I'm down to a crawl. My patience is dying faster than my chemo-poisoned cells. How does one get motivated to run a race one never planned or wanted to enter in the first place?

Although I've never been a natural athlete, I know what it's like to experience the exhilaration of a good run. Before this breast cancer race, in fact, I ran in many freely chosen races.

I close my eyes and visualize myself as a carefree farm-girl, racing my younger brothers and sisters down our long driveway to the waiting school bus. Laughing and panting, I board the bus—being careful not to make eye contact with the patience-challenged driver.

Finding solace in the memory-lane respite from today's tribulations, I allow my closed-eyelid movie-screen to picture me as a college girl. Behind schedule and loaded down with textbooks, I am on one of my regular beat-the-clock sprints to class. Even those races across campus—necessitated by irresponsible time management rather than free choice—held an inherent excitement of sorts.

Now, I am seeing myself in more recent years. After a long day, I'd reward myself by challenging the sun to a race. Feeling healthy and vibrant, I'd run the field road along the creek to my destination—a gravel pit with hill-like mounds. Settling onto a gravel-covered perch atop my favorite miniature mountain, my huffing and puffing, my sweating and stewing, gradually gave way to nature's wonder-working powers.

I bask in the beauty of the fields, homesteads, and distant woods that enhance my panoramic view. I allow the evening breeze to caress my frazzled nerves. My anxieties diminish with the setting sun as it fades over the horizon. Thankful that the sun has allowed me to win the race to the hill before darkness, I begin my walk home.

My reminiscing over, I open my eyes to the present—to the reality of today's race. The stark contrast between my previous races and my cancer race overwhelms me. The race that remains before me looms more dismal then ever.

Jesus knew life would bring unplanned, unwanted races. Jesus knew our patience would at times run low, run out. That's why verse two of the twelfth chapter of Hebrews brings us from running and patience and racing to Jesus and faith. It's our faith muscle that needs to be strengthened, and it is Jesus who has authored and will finish our faith muscle workout.

Today I won't focus on what I can't stand to face even one more day. Instead, I'll choose to face Jesus and ask Him to strengthen my faith.

> **O God, I don't feel like I can run this race any longer. My running energy and patience seem to be exhausted. But I can exercise my free will. Help me look to Jesus, the author and finisher of my faith. I choose to put my faith in**

Jesus and trust Him to run this race with me today and every day until I cross the finish line. Thank you, Lord, for never running out of patience with me, but instead giving Your Son to help me not only finish my race but also to strengthen my faith. Amen.

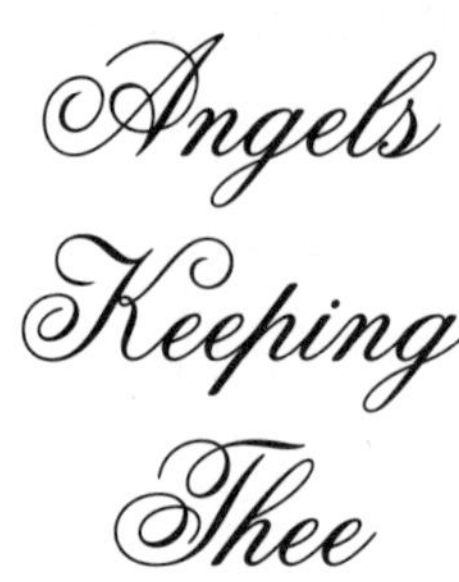

For He shall give His angels charge over thee, to keep thee in all thy ways.
—Psalm 91:11 (KJV)

The small padded envelope arrived in the mailbox along with the junk mail of the day. Perplexed, I opened the envelope and out fell a beautiful delicate angel. Upon closer examination, I recognized it as a duplicate of the angel pin worn by my friend Maxine.

Maxine and I had been acquaintances for years, but our relationship evolved into a friendship during our similar courses of treatment for breast cancer. While having lunch together a few weeks earlier, I had complimented her on the angel pin she was wearing. Now, because of her thoughtfulness, I too could wear the lovely, feminine, gold-and-pearl angel.

The card attached to the angel pin carried a message: Psalm 91:11. The angel was not only an article of jewelry, but like many of the angels in Scripture it also was a messenger. The back of the card bore an inscription: "Handcrafted With Love By" followed by the name, address, and telephone number of the angel's creators.

I had been trying to think of an appropriate gift to give some of the "angels" who had indeed been used by God to help "keep me in all of my ways" during my breast cancer experience.

Realizing that the angel pin was the perfect gift, I dialed the telephone number printed on the card. The voice that responded to the telephone ring was warm and friendly.

After introducing myself to the woman who answered, I explained why I wanted to order several of the angels. There was a pause and then she said, "I'm a ten-year breast cancer survivor. I'm seventy-five years old and my husband and I find great purpose and satisfaction in handcrafting the angels."

Within minutes this total stranger and I had formed a connection. As we continued to converse, I said, "Often God shows me His 'angels.' Today He has already shown me three: Maxine, the angel pin, and now you."

As I hung up the telephone, I basked in the warmth of the events that had transpired since the arrival of the small padded envelope. The certainty of "He shall give His angels charge over thee, to keep thee in all thy ways" embraced and renewed my being and I felt as carefree and light as . . . an angel.

> **Dear God, You are the creator of heavenly angels, earthly angels, and a husband-wife team who are heeding Your call to create angel pins that carry Your message. Thank You for keeping charge over me in all my ways. Amen.**

No Romance by the Christmas Tree This Year

Many waters cannot quench love, nor will rivers overflow it.
—The Song of Solomon 8:7

Christmas is filled with simple little traditions at our home. As recent empty-nesters, my husband and I have begun a new tradition that lack of privacy had prohibited earlier. Sometime during the holiday season, usually between Christmas and New Year's Day, we light the candles and Christmas tree lights, put on a romantic compact disc, arrange a blanket and pillows on the floor by the tree, and make love.

This year it hadn't happened. I'd hoped it would, but I could never muster up the physical, emotional, and sexual energy to follow through. We decided to take down some of the Christmas decorations ornaments early, in order to ease the task after New Year's Day. As we took down the ornaments, the usual post-Christmas letdown was accompanied by a tinge of regret that we had silently let the new tradition slip.

I recalled this year's holiday-season lovemaking—in our bed rather than by the Christmas tree. It had been unlike that of any previous year. The depth of caring and tenderness my husband had expressed in his loving me—scarred and increasingly hairless body and all—was romantic beyond anything ambiance could lend.

Yes, there is gentle romance found in everyday devotion expressed through the speaking of reassuring words, the simple gesture of holding hands, and lingering embraces. Sexual intimacy doesn't necessarily require fireworks to be fulfilling. Sometimes the afterglow of loving and being loved brings a magic of its own.

Next year we'll resume our lovemaking by the Christmas tree and hold close the memory of this year when—without any of the extra trimmings—cherishing the love we have for each other was a gift from each other and from God.

O God, thank You for this man who loves me without tinsel or ornaments, or candles, or soft music. Thank You for the gift You have given us in each other. Thank You for the hope we have in You for ever-deepening love, romance, and adventure and fun ahead. Amen.

New Year Doldrums

It will come to pass that before they call, I will answer; and while they are still speaking, I will hear.

—Isaiah 65:24

Our long-standing New Year's Day tradition has been to drive to the home of my husband's sister and brother-in-law. The cross-country skiers in the family arrive around 1:00, load up gear, and drive to a nearby trail for a time of invigorating holiday calorie-burning and comraderie. Others arrive by 4:30; and everyone convenes shortly thereafter for a potluck lasagna supper. It's always a happy, festive way to celebrate the first day of the new year—exercising in winter-fresh air and enjoying a delicious meal with extended family.

This first day of the new year I was struggling. The cross-country skiing segment of the annual gathering was cancelled because my husband's sister Pat and I were both out of commission due to our respective breast cancer treatments. I was feeling angry at breast cancer for being such a party pooper.

Still reeling from the side effects of my recent chemo treatment, I didn't really feel up to the potluck supper either. Nevertheless, I was determined not to let cancer rob me of that aspect of the holiday. I halfheartedly prepared my salad and we headed to Mavis and Bruce's home.

Within an hour, I found myself thinking, "I shouldn't have come. People probably feel as awkward around me as I feel out of sync with them." I felt tired, achy, and blah—a sort of "Grinch who stole New Year's Day" feeling.

The lasagna supper with garlic bread, salads, and leftover Christmas goodies added to my melancholy mood. My taste buds were still damaged from the first set of four chemo treatments. Everything on the buffet table looked enticing and flavorful, but lost its appeal and taste as it entered my mouth. Bah, humbug!

I made a lackluster effort to socialize, but my feelings were too tenuous for me to find the conversations satisfying. Oh, I knew it wasn't my in-laws' fault. I was out of kilter; but I couldn't will myself back to normal.

Near tears, I sought out my sister-in-law Shirley, a breast cancer survivor and possible source of support. Immediately sensing my need, she responded with sensitivity and acceptance. Feasting on her compassion and encouragement and her promise to "pray me through" the remaining three chemo treatments, I was nourished in ways beyond the reach of a lasagna supper. Uplifted, I enjoyed the remainder of the family gathering despite my achy body.

Preparing for bed that night, my reflection in the mirror nudged my fragile sense of esteem back on the track of despondency. The longer I studied my image, the more unattractive I felt. I was beginning to loath the fleece nightcap and plaid robe I wore to cover my baldness and scars. What a drastic change from my skimpy, feminine nightwear my husband and I both used to enjoy!

Though my romantic mood on a scale of one to five was in the minus range, we made love. Afterwards, holding back tears, I said, "Thank you."

"What?" my husband's voice questioned through the darkness.

"I said, thank you for being willing to make love to me when I'm so ugly."

He comforted me with embraces and loving words, yet I felt so sad. As I drifted off to sleep, I sensed the hounds of depression were chasing me, catching up to me, nipping at my heels—and I was getting too worn out to outrun them any longer.

The next morning I woke up at 8:30. I was alone in bed. A bit groggy, I remembered Colin had decided to use a personal day on the second of January. The plan was to take down our remaining Christmas decorations together. He was likely to be in the sunroom reading the newspaper while waiting for me to wake up.

I welcomed the time alone to think. "I don't think I can look in the mirror again. I don't think I can cook another tasteless breakfast. I don't think I can get out of bed this morning. I don't think I can get out of bed ever again." I felt like I was sinking and unable to help myself.

Just then, my husband bounded around the corner into our bedroom and pounced down on the bed beside me. Before I could think or feel or speak, he burst forth with, "Let's go out for breakfast!" His unexpected surprise was just what I needed to jolt me out of my de-escalating mood. Even though everything except the orange juice tasted odd, the ambience at the restaurant was cheerful, our server a delight, and our impromptu morning date a total success.

Once home again, we listened to our favorite compact discs while taking down decorations. Then my husband decided we were working much too hard for a vacation day. We left everything and went to a matinee of the new movie version of "The Grinch Who Stole Christmas." Sitting among children, we felt silly and carefree. There would be no "Grinch Who Stole the New Year," starring me, after all!

Dear God, I wasn't recognizing the danger signs of impending depression, but You were. Thank you for coming to help me through Shirley and my husband. Even before I called, You answered. While I was still speaking—with my voice and in my mind—You heard and came to my rescue. I'm so grateful for Your marvelous caregiving. Amen.

Encouragement

Therefore encourage one another, and build up one another.
—I Thessalonians 5:11

Today is the third day of January. My husband returned to his job at school today, following a memorable Christmas–New Year break. He was a tremendous encouragement to me, as he loved me through a holiday season of highs and lows.

It is also a Wednesday—my busy day on weeks I'm not scheduled for a chemotherapy treatment. I am eagerly anticipating the living of this day, though my physical and emotional well being are still a bit tenuous. Almost a week since my first taxol chemotherapy treatment, I'm still feeling uneasy about how the chemical seems to clash with my body chemistry. Though I'm relieved that five of my total regiment of eight chemo treatments are behind me, I'm feeling apprehensive as I ponder the remaining three taxol treatments.

From eight to ten o'clock, I attend a weekly Wednesday morning prayer fellowship. Our hostess's daughter, back from a missionary stint halfway around the world, shares her experiences with us this morning. This young woman, so full of ability and faith, tells of the hunger that her adult refugee students expressed for the Bible and its teachings. Serving the Lord, stretching far beyond her comfort zone, she has chosen a path of challenge. It is obvious that she has grown and been blessed in the process. She inspires and encourages me.

Next, I meet my pastor for our monthly "share-and-prayer" time. Six years ago, he and I began to meet on Wednesday mornings to share our current concerns and to pray for our respective ministries. This Wednesday, however, I need more than a share-and-prayer partner; I need my pastor. As I confide the struggles of the past few days and my brush with depression, my voice chokes and the tears spill down my cheeks. My pastor prays that I will know God's presence, strength, and comfort during times I am "in the crucible." I am encouraged by his intent listening, caring, and prayer. I hope he, in turn, is encouraged as he carried out his calling of serving as a minister to me.

Several blocks away and a few minutes later, I pick up Maxine. I had called her just last night, hoping she could join me during her lunch hour. A few months ahead of me in a similar course of treatment for breast cancer, Maxine has already completed her taxol chemotherapy. I am eager to question her about her experience and tell her about mine. As a taxol veteran, Maxine shares many pearls of wisdom with me. Especially meaningful are the words spoken by her oncologist: "Because every person has his or her own unique body chemistry, no two people respond to taxol or any other type of chemotherapy exactly the same way. There are some established standard side effects, but certainly a range of variation within each recipient."

Even though my body's reaction seems to be more severe than hers, I feel encouraged and prepared to continue with the final three treatments. Perhaps most encouraging is Maxine's countenance—she appears happy, optimistic, and healthy.

My final stop is at the home of our daughter, on maternity leave following the birth of our first grandchild. After placing Hudson in my arms, Krissy bundles up and heads outside for the treat of a solitary walk down their driveway to pick up the mail. I am swept with sentiment as I watch her stride into the distance, temporarily free of maternal duties. I am still adjusting to the reality that my little girl is now a mommy.

Later, with Hudson again nestled and dozing in Krissy's arms, we have a mutually encouraging heart-to-heart talk. We share our concerns and struggles with one another. I wrap my arms around my daughter and her tiny child and pray before I leave. The cleansing tears of love and encouragement flow freely and, like an early spring rain, leave us refreshed, renewed, and ready to resume our responsibilities.

* * *

Driving home now, I realize that I have just experienced a great deal of encouragement. My inner strength and resolve to persevere have been built up. I am reminded of the Apostle Paul's words in First Thessalonians that tell us to "encourage one another, and build up one another." I have experienced a day during which ordinary people blessed me in extraordinary ways by their heeding of Paul's words. I continue on my homeward drive with my heart overflowing with thankfulness and praise.

Dear God, You are the Divine Encourager. I'm grateful that You have created Your children with the capacity to encourage one another through the discouraging times of life. Like mortar holds together bricks, encouragement in the form of a smile, hug, word of counsel, kind deed, embrace, tear, gift, or prayer builds up—not just me, not just the other—but one another. Amen.

Bald Trees, Bald Heads

Then God said, "Let the earth sprout vegetation, plants yielding seed, and fruit trees bearing fruit after their kind, with seed in them, on the earth"; and it was so. And the earth brought forth vegetation, plants yielding seed after their kind and trees bearing fruit, with seed in them, after their kind, and God saw that it was good.

—Genesis 1: 11,12

It is one of those winter-wonderland phenomena that mesmerize the senses. The heavy overnight fog, coupled with a light snowfall, has transformed our rather ugly brown trees of January into a scene of awe-inspiring beauty. Seized by the wonder of the view from our sunroom, I sit on the loveseat, gazing out, unable to divert my eyes from the scene before me.

I know of makeovers for women, but for trees? Yesterday the trees looked drab, bleak, and forlorn in their winter nakedness. This morning they look elegant, ready for a pageant in their dazzling white cloaks.

My mind wanders to my encounter with my own seasonal baldness. Last summer the tree branches were filled with leaves, and I had a full head of hair. As the autumn season commenced, the leaves began to fall, along with my hair. By winter the trees and I were sisters in our baldness.

I know that in the spring the tree buds will appear, followed by tiny and then full-grown leaves. Also in the spring my chemotherapy treatments will be over and my hair will begin to grow again.

But the hope of this morning's majesty is not for springtime, but for today. I could be content in the drabness, the bleakness, the forlornness of my baldness, or I could, like the trees, transform it into something elegant—or fun, or whimsical, or sexy, or anything my imagination permits. A variety of wigs, hats, scarves, caps, turbans, earrings, cosmetics are waiting to transform not only my appearance but also my self-image and mood. Sometimes the wings of dawn surprise the new day with unexpected and beautiful transformations.

O God, during my season of baldness, help me to create beauty out of drabness, adventure out of bleakness, hope out of forlornness. Help me to remember that winter is only a season and is not forever. Spring and its promise of new life is just around the corner. For the wonder of creation and You the Creator, I give praise. Amen.

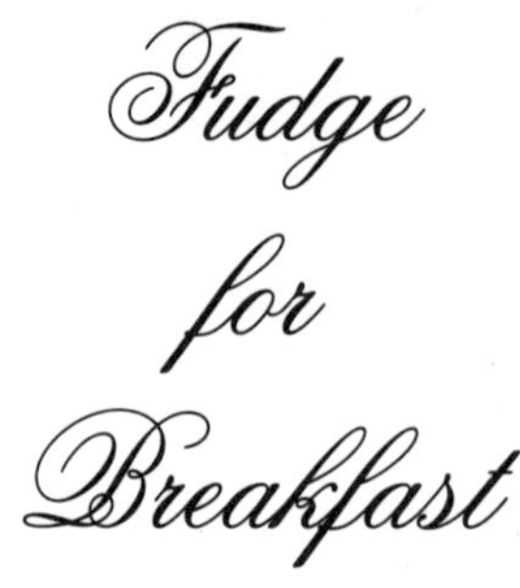

For who can eat and who can have enjoyment without Him?
—Ecclesiastes 2:25

"I don't recall ever having a plate of fudge on our breakfast table before," my husband ventured cautiously. It was December sixth, and my fourth chemotherapy treatment, the last of a series, with its side effect of nausea and appetite loss, was scheduled for that afternoon. An admitted chocoholic and proud of it, my favorite Christmas season delicacy is homemade fudge. Concerned that nausea would prevent me from enjoying the treat later, I had made a batch the night before. We each partook of a piece of fudge as the finale to our breakfast.

After my husband left for work, I devoured a second piece with gusto, then savored a third. After a few moments of contemplating the risk factor to my afternoon chemo treatment, I threw caution to the wind. I daintily reached for the fourth. I wallowed in the exquisite lusciousness, succulence, and decadence of that final piece. With the last morsel melting in my mouth, I allowed myself to linger in the sweet, chocolatey afterglow.

Christmas and New Year's came and went; February was approaching. My taste buds still had not fully recovered from the cumulative effect of the damage incurred by the chemo treatment in early December. That reality, plus the chemical taste in my mouth following the first two treatments in my latest chemo series, had robbed me of the pleasure of eating for any reason other than for needed nourishment. "No, your taste buds have not actually been killed. They will heal eventually," my oncology nurse clinician reassures.

In the meantime, all I have to do is close my eyes and remember my breakfast gala in fudge heaven. That episode taught me to live even the smallest joys of life to the fullest whenever I can—even if it sometimes means breaking through the boundaries of what I deem to be personally or culturally appropriate.

Dear Lord, thank You for creating me with taste buds and a palate to fully enjoy a myriad of food tastes and textures. Forgive me when I so easily take these pleasures for granted until I lose them. Help me to seize little opportunities to break my rules of shoulds and shouldnots so that I may be able to delight in the treats of life. Amen.

Obituaries

Whatever is true, whatever is honorable, whatever is right, whatever is pure, whatever is lovely, whatever is of good repute, if there is any excellence and if anything of praise, let your mind dwell on these things.
—Philippians 4:8

I rarely looked at the obituary pages until after my breast cancer diagnosis. At the time of my diagnosis we were subscribing to the daily newspaper of a large metropolitan area. After scanning the Variety section, comics, advice columnists, and entertainment section, I'd note that the remaining pages were the obituaries and move on to another section of the newspaper.

One day following my diagnosis, however, I paused to scan the obituary pages to see if there were any women near my age. There she was. With her bright eyes and radiant smile, she looked the picture of health—and just a year older than I.

As I proceeded to read the obituary below the picture, I was chilled by the words, "died following a courageous battle with breast cancer." Those words, along with her image, clung like a shadow for the remainder of the day.

During the weeks that followed, I yielded often to the temptation to just take a quick peek at the obituary section. What began as a flirtation was becoming more and more of a daily routine: hunt for a face or age close to mine, then cautiously read the obituary probing for a clue to the cause of death. Almost always the words, "following a courageous battle with breast cancer," or "memorials preferred for breast cancer research," would be there.

I tried to justify this unsettling habit by praying for the listed survivors. As time went on, however, I began to recognize a lingering sadness after reading the obituaries that was becoming increasingly difficult to shake.

While having lunch with a woman who had recently completed her breast cancer treatment, I confessed, "I don't think I should look at the obituary pages any more. They are just too upsetting." She exclaimed, "You've realized that too! I thought it was just me!"

As we talked, we recognized the wisdom and applicability of Philippians 4:8. While experiencing a life-threatening disease, it simply is not healthy or edifying to expose oneself unnecessarily to information about women who have succumbed to that disease. Our world is abounding in uplifting stimuli. Let us partake extravagantly of these.

> **O Lord, every day You bring into my life things that are true, honorable, right, pure, lovely, of good repute, of excellence, and worthy of praise. Open my eyes and ears and mind to dwell on these things so that Your peace will be in me. Amen.**

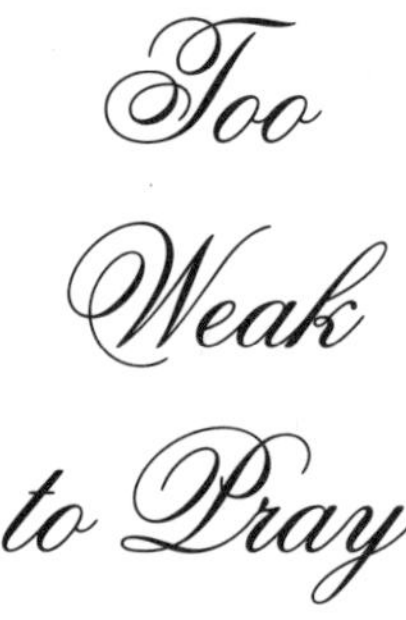

He gives power to the weak, and to those who have no might He increases strength.

—Isaiah 40:29

Today I feel too weak to do anything but exist. Where is the strength that seemed in the past to rarely wane? I lie on my bed too weary to have my daily devotions, to pray for anyone, including myself. I'm thankful the bathroom is close to the bedroom as the prospect of walking a few feet looms like an Olympic marathon. My thoughts turn to my 79-year-old mother, so full of vigor and activity. It is humbling to have less energy than my mother.

I've gathered reading materials for days like today, but even reading lacks appeal. I'm content to just rest, with my eyes open, gazing out the window. An airplane comes into view high in the distance. I visualize it full of people with places to go, things to do. Nearer by, a man and his dog meander down the hiking trail. I can't help but envy their outing on this brisk, sunny, winter morning. A small flock of mourning doves lands to socialize and to peck nourishment from our deck feeder. Even they seem to have more strength than I do.

My recollection of Isaiah 40:29—God's promise to give power to the weak and increased strength to those who have no might—stirs hope within me. Yes, I believe there is power in God's unconditional love, in faith, in hope. Yes, I believe in the truth of Jesus' response when the Apostle Paul, as recorded in 2 Corinthians 12:9, asked three times to have the thorn in his flesh removed: "My grace is sufficient for you, for power is perfected in weakness." Yes, I believe—and for now I am content in that certainty.

Dear Lord, I'm grateful that the days I struggle with physical weakness are only temporary. Even when I feel too weak to pray, I am gently held in the palm of Your hand. I can rest in the assurance that Your grace, strength, and power are sufficient for today. Thank you. Amen.

Grandchild Therapy

Like a shepherd He will tend His flock, in His arms He will gather the lambs, and carry them in His bosom: He will gently lead the nursing ewes.
—Isaiah 40:11

One of God's most precious blessings during my cancer journey has been the birth of our first grandchild. My surgery phase of treatment coincided with our daughter Krissy's third trimester of pregnancy. We bonded in new ways as mother-daughter chats often turned to the trials and joys of surgeries and pregnancy. With my second surgery scheduled at the same hospital where our grandchild would be delivered, we realized we could possibly be in the hospital at the same time and hoped that would not be the case. It wasn't.

Hudson Kenneth, a gentleman from the start, postponed his debut a full fifteen days, allowing his novice grandma to be sufficiently recovered and prepared to be on hand for his arrival. Further, God provided me with the needed strength to stay with the new little family of three for the first week, as planned, to assist with meals and moral support.

My first chemotherapy treatment was two weeks after Hudson's birth. Throughout my five months of chemotherapy, I was able to spend time with Hudson for a day or two almost every week. This little person, so innocent and fresh from God's hand of creation, has been able to provide a healing therapy that is beyond the skills of a medical professional.

Hudson and I, grandmother and grandson, are years apart in age and life experience, and yet we have so much in common. The visible kinship is that we are both baldies! We are both of fragile strength and in need of daytime naps. I often fall asleep with him in my arms as we snuggle into the safe embrace of the big soft recliner. We both have our physical frustrations. Hudson has his gas pains and more recently the onset of teething pain. I had my nausea discomfort during the first set of chemo treatments and now my muscle aches for the second. Sometimes I feel like crying, and Hudson cries for both of us.

But beyond the cuddling and sleeping and crying has been my week-by-week sharing in the emergence of Hudson's distinct personality. This child is more than a body; he is also a soul and a spirit. God created Hudson in my daughter's womb as she had been created by God in mine and I in my mother's. I realize that God has a special plan for this child, as for all children, and I am privileged to be a part of that plan. Although I am now a grandmother, I am also God's precious child; and His plan for my life is still unfolding. Just as Hudson's infant body is held close to my scarred bosom, we both are held close to the bosom of our Creator. As in Isaiah 40:11, God is our shepherd, tending to us both, gathering us as His lambs, and carrying us in His bosom.

Dear Shepherd, Thank You for creating and loving us as Your beloved lambs. Whether a babe fresh from a mother's womb or a woman cradling her child's child, we are carried in the nurture of Your bosom throughout our lives. Thank You for Your tender care. Amen.

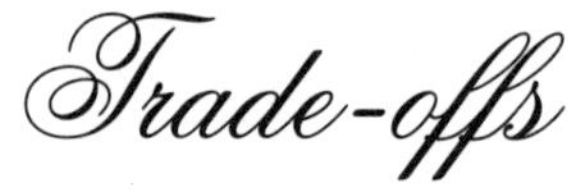

Thou hast turned for me my mourning into dancing; Thou hast loosed my sackcloth and girded me with gladness.

—Psalm 30:11

The most bittersweet times during my breast cancer journey were the missed once-in-a-lifetime occasions. Those times were bitter when my physical condition prohibited my sharing in the celebrations, yet sweet in the unique blessings that were substituted.

My nephew Luke's wedding to his beloved Darcie was on the Saturday following my Wednesday surgery. When my surgery date was set, I'd informed my surgeon of the wedding date. He was confident I would be up to attending.

What neither of us had anticipated, however, was my difficult recovery from the anesthesia. My sister Carol, a nurse, called on Friday to see how I was doing. After I mournfully confided how I was *really* feeling, she advised, "Listen to your body in making your decision tomorrow."

Saturday morning my body was still feeling worn out and faint. With a heavy heart, I called my mother to inform her that I wasn't yet up to the drive and wedding. Colin and I would be staying home. "The wedding will be videotaped," she consoled me. She and others in attendance would tell us all about it later.

It turned out to be one of those rare perfect July days in Minnesota—sunny, with a fresh gentle breeze and ideal temperature. "A perfect day for a wedding," I said, sighing in disappointment.

It was also a perfect day to rest outdoors, I decided, and I proceeded to set up a chaise lounge by our landscaped waterfall and shade garden. The unflawed peacefulness and beauty of the setting became my healing balm as the afternoon unfolded—the sun filtering through the tree canopy, the singing birds sipping their fill from the still pool above the falling stream, the ripple of the water. Mandy, our German shepherd dog, and Midnight, the cat, sauntered over and curled by my side for a lazy snooze.

At mid-afternoon my husband took a break from this unexpected gift of time that he was using to putter around the yard, and brought out two glasses of icy lemonade. We had labored hard to design and complete this serene haven two summers before, but this was the first day we actually sat down long enough to bask in the fruit of our labor.

Later my husband's brother Bill saw me as he drove by and pulled in to chat. Soon after, his wife, Shirley, a breast cancer survivor, came to be my companion and encourager. The day turned out to be one of my happiest ever.

* * *

Aunt Mona was 104 when she died in November. The funeral service was to be a grand celebration of her long life. Though Mona was my husband's aunt, I loved and admired her and I ached with mourning—especially when I realized the low white cell count and extreme fatigue that followed my most recent chemotherapy treatment would prohibit me from attending the service.

Instead, I set aside the afternoon of her funeral and simultaneously held a personal service of memorial in our sunroom. I had a copy of the funeral bulletin, so I prayed for the various portions of the service, sang the hymns solo, and reflected on my memories of Mona. I'd asked my husband to audio-tape the service, which proved to be a blessing, not only to me but also to out-of-state relatives who had not been able to attend. Indeed, God turned my mourning into dancing!

* * *

My mother-in-law's ninety-second birthday was celebrated on a January Sunday. The side effects from my second set of chemotherapy treatments included muscle aches and weakness, particularly in my legs. I was simply too uncomfortable to attend the morning church service honoring her or the afternoon birthday party.

What was the trade-off? By Wednesday I felt fine and brought lunch to her at home for a private after-the-party celebration. As she bubbled over with joy in telling me who had come, describing the cake, and showing me her gifts, I realized how honored I was to be having her all to myself. My heart was filled with gladness!

Dear Lord, I'm so grateful that You are able to turn missed opportunities into lasting blessings. You are the One who turns mourning and disappointment into dancing and gladness. You are the One I trust and praise. Amen.

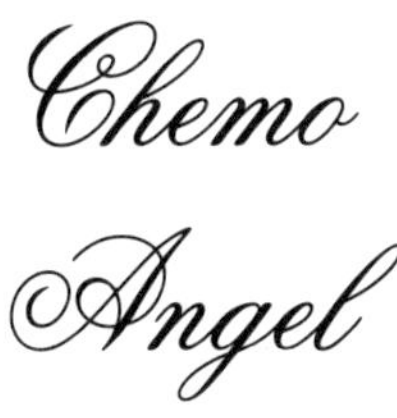

Chemo Angel

And it will also come to pass that before they call, I will answer.
—Isaiah 65:24

God chose Evelyn to be my angel during the almost six-month trek through chemotherapy. Before I had even recognized the need for a companion, Evelyn approached me after a church service and offered to sit with me during my upcoming chemotherapy treatments. Overwhelmed by the generosity of her offer, I was pleased to accept. I doubt that either of us recognized at the time that this was a holy encounter arranged by God Himself.

My husband was with me for two of my eight treatments; Evelyn was there for the others. Just minutes into our first session together, a beautiful embroidery project made its first of six appearances. "This is a pillow cover I'm making for a dear friend in the Ukraine," Evelyn casually explained.

I was aware that Evelyn and her husband, George, had been on short-term mission trips to a sister church in Ukraine and that the next planned visit was forthcoming. As I lethargically glanced at the handwork draped over Evelyn's lap, I noted the loveliness of the blue-and-rose floral pattern that she was stitching on an ivory backround.

Drip by drip, stitch by stitch, the chemotherapy sessions progressed. Evelyn proved an engrossing conversationalist. She held my rapt attention. I was inspired not only by her missions to Ukraine but also by her ministry with teenage girls and church women, her dedication to George and their family, her caring for neighbors, her varied hobbies—she even shared a recipe with me for raspberry truffles. There was a bubbling over of the joy and wisdom of Jesus that I progressively took care to glean as Evelyn stitched and chatted.

Enlightenment came just after my seventh treatment as I rested and pondered my now-waning chemotherapy experience. While the drip, drip of the toxic chemicals entering my veins was accomplishing the purposed destruction of something ugly, the stitch, stitch of Evelyn's needle was simultaneously creating something beautiful. Yes, Evelyn was chosen by God to bring something to the chemotherapy room beyond conversation and companionship. Through the beauty, joy, and purpose she was stitching into a love gift bound for Ukraine, God was revealing triumph over disease and hope for the future; indeed, a future so full of life and hope that I too could dream of a mission trip someday—perhaps even a rendezvous with this blue, rose, and ivory pillow-cover in the home of a faraway Ukrainian woman.

Dear Lord, Your angels come to this earth in many places and forms. Thank You for the one who came to a chemotherapy room to deliver Your message of beauty, love, and hope through the stitches of an embroidery needle. Help us to recognize the earthly angels You bring to us and the messages You deliver through them. Amen.

The Last Chemo: Farewell Thoughts

He has brought me to his banquet hall, and his banner over me is love.
—Song of Solomon 2:4

Tomorrow will be my last chemotherapy treatment, the day I have been looking forward to ever since my surgeon first informed me of my need for chemotherapy. It is the day I began to anticipate even more after my oncologist recommended adding taxol to my treatment plan, expanding the number of total sessions from four to eight; the day I often thought would never come. But it is actually coming. It will be tomorrow.

For five months my life has revolved around the rhythm of the twenty-one-day chemotherapy treatment cycle—blood tests, chemo treatment, forty-eight hours of expelling chemicals, dealing with side effects, rebounding, and going back to repeated blood tests.

With the yearned-for finish in sight, I contemplate the trek I have been on. While I do so, a Scripture song I learned years ago drifts through my mind. Recalling that the song came from Song of Solomon 2:4, I flip through my Bible to read the verse anew: "He has brought me to his banquet hall, and his banner over me is love." This seems an unlikely verse to relate to my treatment experience. It is difficult to imagine a chemotherapy room as a banquet hall. One hardly thinks of intravenous feeding of toxic chemicals as a feast. And where is the banner of love?

Now, with fresh insight, God enables me to view the chemotherapy experience in a new light. It has not been just chairs, and bags of toxic chemicals, IV tubes, and a clock. It has also been Annette, my oncology nurse clinician. At first I viewed Annette only as the medical professional associated with the dreaded treatments. As the sessions progressed, our conversations evolved from polite chit-chat to sharing tidbits about our personal lives and to a sense of mutual respect and caring. We each have a life beyond the chemotherapy room that includes a husband, children, home, church, relatives, and more.

During a recent session, I asked Annette why she chose to become an oncology nurse clinician. With her answer came my realization that this is not just a job to Annette. She cares about what she is doing and each person for whom she is doing it. Her genuine caring is evident in her conscientious professional performance, her offering of helpful resources, her cheerful willingness to provide copies of my lab tests, and her answering my many questions patiently and thoughtfully.

Annette said, "One of the things I find difficult, though, is not seeing my patients after their treatments end and wondering how they are doing." Her statement has lingered in my mind and now illuminates the relevance of Song of Solomon 2:4.

Yes, although a paradox, the chemotherapy room I have been coming to these many months is indeed a banquet hall of healing. And yes, the banner over me was and is love. And yes, I will be back from time to time to greet Annette and to tell her how I am doing.

I sense that I will sleep well tonight. Whether my final chemotherapy treatment tomorrow will bring forth shouts of jubilation, feelings of melancholy, or tears of relief, I am secure in the care of God and the healers He has provided for me.

Dear Great Physician, thank You for bringing me safely to the eve before my last chemotherapy treatment. Thank You also for the

Annettes of this world who use their training and gifts as a part of Your healing team. I'm grateful for their dedication and hard work, their willingness to juggle personal and professional lives, and their caring and compassion. Thank You for the banner of love that is over me and over others who are brought to the chemotherapy banquet hall. Amen.

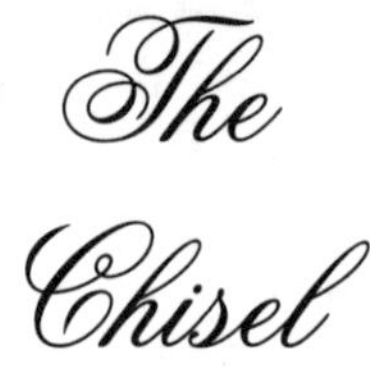

Thy hands made me and fashioned me; give me understanding, that I may learn Thy commandments.
—Psalm 119:73

As I hurried to accept my package and head to the door of the Christian bookstore, my eyes were diverted for a moment to a print on display. I stopped abruptly, pulled toward the image. Like a fish lured by tantalizing bait, I allowed myself to be hooked and reeled in to the display table.

Enthralled, I studied the print. It was a painting of a man's upper body being chiseled by the hand of God. Observing the man's chest, arms, and hands, I saw that he appeared to be strong, muscular, healthy—seemingly to the degree that he could have pushed away the chisel and the hand that was guiding it. But no, the man was in the posture of submission with his shoulders bent slightly forward and his hands passively clasped. My eyes moved upward to study his face. The artist had skillfully created indistinct features—the face could be that of any man.

What transcended features was facial expression. The man was obviously in pain, was suffering under the pressure of the chisel. Yet, it was clear that he was choosing to endure rather than fight or flee.

"Why?" I wondered. His muscled physique revealed he had experienced the "no pain, no gain" creed associated with body-building training. Perhaps now he was ready to endure the pain necessary to move beyond building body strength to building character strength. Perhaps his free will had brought him to the realization that the Master Chiseler could accomplish what the man in his own power could not. Perhaps he desired to be the best man he could be and was willing to trust the Chiseler to bring about the intended masterpiece.

* * *

"Am I, too, being chiseled?" I ponder. I didn't choose a breast cancer experience to serve as a chisel. But—maybe the man in the painting didn't initially choose to be chiseled, either. At some point, he opened his free will to the chisel, trusting that the end result would be worth the temporary pain.

What is being chiseled from me? I don't yet see the sculpted masterpiece, but I do see some of the fragments that have fallen. One is shallow empathy for others who are enduring illness or other difficulties. Yes, the chisel is bringing forth within me an ever-deepening characteristic of compassion.

Another fragment is self-pride in my perception of being healthy and physically fit, along with a subtle negative attitude and impatience toward those who aren't. Now I view health and fitness not only as the result of my own effort but also as a gift of God's grace.

Stubborn independence is yet another fragment that has fallen victim to the chisel. I realize now that I need other people. I need the prayers, love, support, wisdom, encouragement, companionship, practical assistance, medical care, and more that God channels through others. Though the chiseling is not yet complete, I need not fear the chisel because it is unerring in the hand of the Divine Chiseler. I am invited to submit to the process in faith that I am becoming a better, more fulfilled woman because of it.

O God, help me to trust Your gentle, loving hand as You allow this breast cancer experi-

ence to be a chisel—not to break or destroy, but rather to create in me Your masterpiece. Please give me the understanding, patience, and faith I need during this process. Amen.

Radiation Treatment and Recovery

Valentine's Day Requests

Delight yourself in the Lord; and He will give you the desires of your heart.
—Psalm 37:4

"What would you like for Valentine's Day?" I asked my husband at the breakfast table on February 14. Hesitantly, he ventured, "How about a simple meal here at home . . . and maybe you could wear your rose negligee."

After thirty-three years of marriage, it took only a split second of eye contact for me to know that my husband had put a lot of forethought into his request. He knew the desire of his heart and was asking for it.

I paused to ponder what granting his request would entail. It would mean setting a formal table in our dining room, some creative decorating, serving the easy-to-prepare chicken cashew casserole he favors, and maybe even hors d'oeuvres and a glass of wine in the sunroom beforehand. And the rose negligee? The *transparent* rose negligee? Flashing the most romantic 6:30 in the morning smile I could muster, I replied, "You've got it!"

Once my husband left for work, I hurried to get ready for my 8:30 until 11:00 appointment at the Radiology Treatment Center. Although my final chemotherapy treatment was two weeks away, I was scheduled to begin the preliminaries today for the upcoming radiation phase of breast cancer treatment. I didn't have many clues what to expect.

As the morning at the treatment center progressed, I was measured for my protective lead alloy molds, experienced a simulation run-through, and had a computerized tomography scan. I tried valiantly to absorb the new terminology and technology and to lie perfectly still during the various procedures.

I forgot about my husband's Valentine's Day request until I noticed that the right side of my chest had acquired an array of ugly, black felt-tip pen markings. The thirty-something male technician was placing wide strips of transparent tape over the marks and explaining, "These markings are made with permanent marker, but I'm putting tape over them to make sure they don't wash off before your next appointment." He must have read the dismay in my eyes, because he continued, "You don't have a problem with that, do you?"

Feeling a bit vulnerable and foolish lying on the table, bare from the waist up except for my black marks and transparent tape strips, I blurted out my husband's Valentine's Day request. "If this was any day but Valentine's Day, I wouldn't care . . . but I don't think my husband had black marks and tape strips in mind when he said he hoped I'd wear my transparent negligee tonight."

Blushing a rosier rose than my soon-to-be worn negligee, the technician walked to a cabinet and returned with a handful of small packets. Handing them to me, he said with a wink, "It's too long to expect you to keep these marks intact anyway. Just peel the tape off and use these cleaning pads to remove the marks. I'll re-mark when you come in for your next appointment." As I left the room, he smiled and said, "You two have a great Valentine's Day!"

Catching my reflection in the rearview mirror as I drove home, I noted a quirky grin on my face. I was thinking about the unusual forms cupid can take. This Valentine's Day, our cupid took the form of a radiation technician! I imagined him going home after work and exclaiming to his wife, "Do you know that people over fifty still have a romantic sex life? Even women over fifty who are being treated for breast cancer still have a romantic sex life!" Perhaps, in some strange way, I, in return, would be their cupid.

It was a special, memorable Valentine's Day evening. Returning home from my appointment inspired, I reached to the back of my intimate apparel drawer. Retrieving the lacy panties and bras I hadn't worn since my diagnosis, I arranged them in a colorful trail from our entry to the sunroom. My husband chuckled as he literally picked up the path leading to our hors d'oeuvres tray. There he found me, his Number One valentine, waiting in my transparent rose negligee.

Oh, there were scars under the negligee; but compared to ugly, black markings and strips of tape, they seemed almost invisible. Besides, we were too busy delighting ourselves in the desires of our hearts to notice. Our Valentine's Day requests were being granted.

Dear God, You are perfect love. Thank You for creating Your children with the capacity to delight in each other. Open our hearts to Your lavish love. Help us to follow Your example in giving each other the desires of our hearts. Amen.

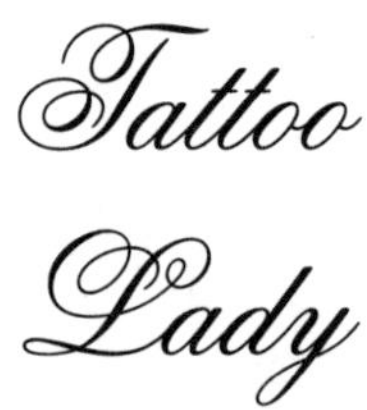

Tattoo Lady

"Can a woman forget her nursing child, and have no compassion on the son of her womb? Even these may forget, but I will not forget you. Behold, I have inscribed you on the palms of my hands."

—Isaiah 49:15,16

Tattoos have always intrigued me. When I was a child, I would occasionally spot someone with a tattoo and stare to the point of causing my parents embarrassment. The person with the tattoo was usually a man who had acquired it while in the military service—an eagle, a heart that proclaimed "I love Mom," or the name of a girlfriend. Sometimes I would further complicate the situation by asking why the name of the woman whom the tattoo proclaimed would be loved forever was not the same as the name of the tattoo-wearer's wife.

After becoming a volunteer at an all-male federal prison several years ago, I studied with interest the tattoos that pattern the skin of some of the inmates who participated in our chapel outreach. Most of the tattoo designs showed fearsome creatures—dragons and various beasts that embellished the full length of the arms. As the inmates came to know and trust Jesus as Lord and Savior, they often expressed regret pertaining to the nature of their tattoos and discussed having them removed eventually.

In recent years, tattoos have become popular with the general population in the United States. Even women of my age sport a tattoo such as small flowers or butterflies on an ankle, breast, buttock, or elsewhere. Temporary tattoos—painted on the face at a carnival or special festivity—and purchased transfers are popular with children. Whether permanent or temporary, it seems that tattoos are often worn as a proclamation or as an enhancement of individual identity.

⁂

This evening as I prepare for bed, I study my own newly acquired "mapping" with amusement and realize that this is probably the closest I'll ever come to being a tattooed lady. Today I went to the Radiation Treatment Center for my block simulation—another preparation step prior to my first real radiation treatment. The medical professional carefully measured and marked and recorded my measurements—all part of a stringent planning procedure ensuring that my radiation treatment will be individualized and accurate. Wide strips of transparent tape were placed over the simplistic tattoo-like markings to prevent them from being washed off in the shower. On some patients, I was told, small permanent needle markings are prescribed.

Hmm—the dark green "tattoos" resemble a plus sign between my breasts and minus signs a few inches to each side. My tattoos are certainly not creative, artistic, beautiful, or even cute. However, like most tattoos, they do serve the purpose of extending personal identity. I am a woman undergoing radiation treatment for breast cancer. I will be reminded of this identity each time I look at my nude chest for the next seven weeks.

Now I think of Isaiah 49:15,16 and visualize my name inscribed on the palms of God's hands—not a temporary wash-off name but a permanently inscribed one. I imagine God looking at my name and identifying me, not as a radiation patient for seven weeks, but as His beloved daughter forever. God promises He will not forget me, but instead will have even more compassion for me than a mother has for her child. I am at peace with who I am and Whose I am.

Dear God, seven weeks with tattoos on my radiated breast seem very brief compared to Your remembering me all of my life and throughout eternity. I'm so grateful that my true identity is established by You—now and forevermore. Amen.

Radiation Treatment: Day One

For we do not have a high priest who cannot sympathize with our weaknesses, but one who has been tempted in all things as we are, yet without sin. Let us therefore draw near with confidence to the throne of grace, that we may receive mercy and find grace to help in time of need.

—Hebrews 4:15,16

I've just arrived home from my first radiation treatment. Everything went smoothly. The drive there and back was uneventful. The receptionist was welcoming. The waiting room was pleasant. The professional staff was friendly and competent. The treatment itself was brief, painless, lacking in trauma.

Why then did I rush to the exit door with such urgency? Why was I so relieved to be within the safe haven of my car? Why was the door barely closed before I collapsed into sobs?

* * *

"Lord," I ask in confusion, "What's going on here?" My head and my heart feel heavy and sad as I reconstruct the day in my mind. I begin speaking aloud to Jesus, my confidant. "My day began with a marvelous gift—the opportunity to audit a course from a previous favorite professor. I thanked you, Lord, as I drove away from the campus. It is as though you've orchestrated my Mondays—every week of my radiation treatment begins with this uplifting learning experience.

"Yes, it was at the radiation treatment center that my happy disposition began to wane. As I attempt to visualize the events of the forty-five minutes between arrival and departure, I ask you to bring into focus the reasons for my struggle.

"Hmmm . . . for two weeks I have been totally free of medical appointments, experiencing only slight aftereffects from my completed chemotherapy treatments. Entering the radiation treatment center thrust me back into reality—I am still a woman being treated for breast cancer.

"My brief flirtation with identifying myself among the healthy people was burst, like a bubble pricked prematurely. No, I was not one of the healthy people in the waiting room—there as drivers or companions. I was a patient. The loss of my identity as a woman full of health and vitality was revisited and it felt like a scab being ripped off a healing wound.

"My grieving was reinforced following the treatment. One of the professional staff informed me that she would be leaving for Florida and someone else would be filling in for her. A form of claustrophobia set in as I realized the necessity of remaining within driving distance of this treatment center for the next seven weeks. Someone else filling in for me would not be an option!

"The final blow came as I was leaving the treatment room. I noticed a wall of cubicles, each the receptacle for a patient's lead alloy block, used to protect vital organs from the potentially damaging radiation. As if entering a time capsule, my mind was transported back twenty-five years to a similar wall I observed while touring the Mayo Clinic. The guide pointed to the wall and soberly explained that each block represented a cancer patient. I vividly recalled my thought at the time: those poor people. Now I was identified with the people I had pitied.

"And now, I am in awe of how You have brought clarity and understanding over these past minutes. You are my Divine listener and counselor. Already my heavy mood is lifting, as I again find inner peace in the assurance of Your abiding care and grace."

* * *

It's been good to permit myself this dance with grief, but now I choose a new partner—gratitude. I'm grateful for the advances in radiation treatment over the past twenty-five years. I'm grateful for the ongoing support of many people. I'm especially grateful to be God's child.

> **Dear Lord, I'm so grateful that I can come with confidence to Your throne of grace to receive mercy and find grace to help me in my times of need. It is a blessing to be able to bare my heart and soul to You as my most intimate confidant, and to know that You are able and willing to listen, guide, and heal. Amen.**

Adapting

For God hath not given us the spirit of fear; but of power, and of love, and of a sound mind.

—2 Timothy 1:7 (KJV)

It is the third day of my radiation treatment and I am feeling quite smug. "I've got this new routine down pat already," I think proudly to myself. The freeway and city streets, as well as the secret code to lift the arm at the entrance to the treatment center parking lot, don't seem as daunting as they did just two days ago.

There is a growing familiarity with the receptionists and the sign-in procedure, the layout, and amenities of the waiting room. I have figured out which people in the waiting room are the patients and which are the drivers and companions.

When my name is called, I know which direction to walk after passing through the double doors. I know where to hang my coat at the entrance to the treatment room. I know I'm to walk across the room to the privacy screen and disrobe from the waist up. I've observed that the stack of clean hospital gowns offers several light blue designs to choose from. I know that I'll take the topmost gown and wear it with the opening to the back.

Centering my body on the table and positioning my head on the contoured headrest seem second nature now. I tuck my left hand under my thigh, just far enough in to keep my arm from slipping off the table. My right arm seems to automatically find its way to the elevated stirrup. The lead alloy block marked with my name and uniquely formed to protect my heart and lung is inserted into the radiation apparatus.

The two technicians carefully check positions and measurements; then they leave the room. Entering the adjacent control center, they carry out their mission. They convey calm confidence as they apply their expertise in activating the machine known as Linear Accelerator—the machine that will quietly perform its ominous task of destroying any residual cancer cells in my breast region.

I lie perfectly still, waiting for the machine's movements and sounds that, though growing in familiarity, are still mysterious to me. I silently pray that God will be in ultimate control of the process. I gaze at the illuminated nature scene on the ceiling above me, lit only on the left side because the light bulb on the right side isn't functioning. The scene on the left side is picturesque and beckoning—vivid foliage and flowers in a mountainous terrain. I hope the bulb on the right will be replaced soon, so I'll be able to view the complete panorama. I listen to the soft, soothing background music, knowing that this wait will be short.

The distinct sound alerting me to the activated machine heightens the senses within my prostrate body. I realize that the radiation is now skimming next to the side of my lung and am careful to follow the technician's directive, "Just breathe normally and don't move." I wonder why I consistently develop an itch on my face and the urge to take a deep breath at this critical juncture. The machine moves to the other side of my breast region and repeats its distinctive drone.

When motion ceases and silence fills the room, I wait just a moment or two for the technicians to return to the room announcing, "You're done!" The elevated table lowers. I hop off and walk the few steps to the changing area. Slipping off my hospital gown, I toss it toward the nearby laundry receptacle. "That's three for three," I congratulate myself on my uncharacteristic athletic prowess.

Yes, I've come a long way since being enveloped by a wave of sadness on my first day of radiation treatment. I am pleased with how quickly I have accepted radiation treatment into my life. I am at peace within my world again.

Dear Lord, thank You for helping me to adapt to this new routine and this phase of treatment. I pray that You will protect and guide every aspect of every treatment and that You will bless the relationships formed during the seven-week duration. Thank You for helping me overcome my spirit of fear, and for replacing it with a spirit of power, and of love, and of a sound mind. Amen.

Strangers at the Gate

And he answered and said, "You shall love the Lord your God with all your heart . . . and your neighbor as yourself." But wishing to justify himself, he said to Jesus, "And who is my neighbor?"

—Luke 10:27,29

The twenty-eighth of thirty-five radiation treatments has taken place today. Now into my sixth week of the 2:00 to 2:15 P.M., Monday-through-Friday appointments, the routine had become rather mundane. Today, because of my boredom with the predictable, I was primed to experience something out of the ordinary. Although I hadn't articulated a prayer to that end, God knew my heart and answered in an amazing way before I even entered the treatment building.

My spiritual adventure—clothed in the guise of the familiar radiation-treatment pattern—began when I approached the entrance gate of the parking lot. As I punched the May code number that prompted the crossbar to raise, another patient punched the exit crossbar button, synchronizing our passing within inches of one another. We exchanged glances, smiles, and slight waving gestures.

The image of the exiting patient remained in my mind as I drove into a parking spot. It was then that God nudged me out of my conditioned complacency and into a keener awareness of what had just occurred.

This wasn't the first time I had seen this particular patient. I had noticed the woman, one among several current radiation patients, a few times before—sometimes in the waiting room, sometimes walking to her car, sometimes alone in an examining room I'd pass while I was being escorted to an adjacent room.

We had never been close enough in proximity to converse, yet I had noticed and admired her choice of clothing, especially her matching trench coat and hat. She had obviously lost her hair during chemotherapy, too, and had apparently opted for hats and scarves rather than a wig. While we had passed each other at the gate today, I'd noticed the scarf she was wearing—a colorful plaid—and had thought she looked attractive wearing it.

We were strangers at the gate. Strangers? She, like me, is so much more than a covered, bald head and a body in need of radiation treatment. She, like me, has come from someplace before arriving at this parking lot and has a destination when she leaves. We both are juggling the responsibilities and activities of our lives to accommodate our treatment schedule. We both are watching clocks and gas tanks and traffic patterns to ensure our timely arrival. We both have people who know and care about our health crisis. We both hope to feel well, and to be healthy in the future. We both have been changed forever by the events that have led to our passing at the gate.

Strangers? No. The knowing glance, smile, and wave affirm our sisterhood. We are both beloved daughters of the Great Physician, kindred travelers down the path of healing, and partakers in this precious gift known as life.

Dear Lord, help me to see the people whose radiation treatment schedules coincide with mine as more than just anonymous patients. Help me to see each one as Your son or daughter. Our paths, as we travel through life, will

cross for just this brief time. Help me to be Your smile, Your word of encouragement, Your messenger of cheer, Your listening ear, or Your waving hand while I am able. These strangers, too, are my neighbors. Help me to love these neighbors as myself. Amen.

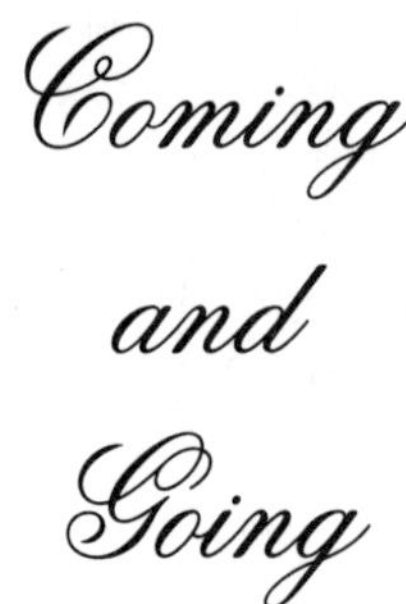

The Lord will guard your going out and your coming in from this time forth and forever.

—Psalm 121:8

Come and go, come and go, come and go. That's what we radiation patients do during the course of our treatment. My treatment prescription is thirty-five "come and go" visits—every Monday, Tuesday, Wednesday, Thursday, and Friday for seven weeks.

Up and down, up and down, up and down. The entrance and exit crossbars in and out of the treatment center parking lot maintain their push-button programmed rhythm as we patients come and go.

Open and shut, open and shut, open and shut. The double doors to the waiting room and the treatment area corridor respond to our push, allowing our coming and going.

In and out, in and out, in and out. We patients walk into the treatment room, undergo our radiation treatment, and walk out.

Undress and dress, undress and dress, undress and dress. The daily routine is quickly learned—disrobe from the waist up, slip on the hospital gown, receive the treatment for the day, remove the hospital gown, and dress.

Into position, out of position, into position, out of position, into position, out of position. The exact position is critical—lie with head and body in position, adjust position to the dictates of precise measurements, remain still in perfect position during treatment, move out of position.

Come and go, up and down, open and shut, in and out, dress and undress, into position, out of position. One envisions a scenario of robots! Indeed, it would be easy for us radiation treatment patients to slip into a state of feeling less than human as the days and then the weeks mechanically march by.

What is the key to protecting and nurturing personal dignity and individuality during the course of such a potentially dehumanizing routine? I am experiencing that key—that safeguard—to be the heart-and-soul connection between the human beings involved in the treatment process.

It exists in the smile, the greeting, and the brief exchange of small talk with the receptionist prior to signing in each day.

The key is present in the waiting room whenever people acknowledge one another instead of merely sitting side by side watching television or paging through the newspaper or magazines.

Even a few words or a knowing nod carries the potential to transcend the sterile production line setting and to shout, "We are unique, marvelous human beings here! We each have a profound personal history, relationships, gifts, worries, and dreams. Each one of us is living an ongoing life story that is only temporarily pausing at this page. *Who* we are matters."

The key appears in the treatment and examining rooms through the staff who hold a power far greater than that of the machines they operate and the technical and medical information they communicate. They hold the capability to enhance or deflate the often-fragile sense of dignity and worth of each patient they encounter.

The safeguarding heart-and-soul connection is played out in the staff members' courtesy of welcoming each patient by name, by the valuing of privacy while each patient is undressing and dressing, and by their offering a few moments of friendly chit-chat while readying for the treatment. It happens when they are able to communicate through their attentiveness: "You and your well-being are important to me and are worthy of my utmost diligence." It is felt when they perceive each patient as not merely a time slot, but as a person loved and valued by God and others—a person very much like them.

Dear Divine Healer, I'm grateful that You created human beings with the ability to construct buildings, develop machines, and learn all that is necessary to make radiation treatments possible. I thank You also for the people You've enabled to work in the field of radiation oncology. They serve as the heart and soul of radiation treatment. I ask You to bless and guide each of them. Amen.

Final Radiation Treatment: What Now?

Those who sow in tears shall reap with joyful shouting. He who goes to and fro weeping, carrying his bag of seed, shall indeed come again with a shout of joy, bringing his sheaves with him.

—Psalms 126:5-6

My final radiation treatment—number thirty-five—is this afternoon. I'm almost giddy with anticipation. Fantasy thoughts race into the near future as I imagine myself cheering "Hallelujah," hugging the radiation therapy technicians in unbridled exuberance, and shouting, "It's over! It's finally over!" to passersby as I head home.

The deep yearning I have harbored since my diagnosis day will finally be fulfilled: my life will be normal again. With adrenaline pumping through my system and my foot heavy on the car's accelerator, I speed to the radiation therapy center for this last treatment. In less than an hour—by 2:30—I will be able to close the breast cancer chapter in my life story and move on. Thankfully, the seat belts will restrain me from doing flips and cartwheels during the drive back home.

* * *

Back in the car now, I'm too limp and bewildered to turn the ignition key. Although my mind feels muddled, I'm able to note the time on the dashboard clock. It is indeed 2:30. As my tears flow, I try desperately to regain composure. The lofty, dramatic visions of joyful shouting have been overtaken by a void that feels almost catatonic.

I try to reconstruct my final radiation treatment in an attempt to figure out what went wrong. When and how were my expectations of jubilation crushed? My starry-eyed aura followed me from the car to the waiting room and lingered during the treatment; but somehow, it remained on the treatment table as I arose to step down for the last time.

Behind the privacy curtain, as I removed the hospital gown and dressed once more, a great void rose up within me and forced out—not a shout—but tears. I tried to muster up my anticipated outpouring of celebration, but the only outpouring that emerged was that of more tears.

Regaining control of my emotions, I stepped out from behind the curtain. Feeling awkward, I said my good-byes to Ken, my radiation therapy technician, and received his good wishes. Instead of skipping merrily away, I found myself turning back for a hug. Choking back what I sensed could be a torrent of tears, I allowed Sue, another of my radiation therapy technicians, to put her arm around me as she guided me to the office of the department head.

"I can't believe this is happening," I croaked, embarrassed and sensing the need to offer an explanation for my bizarre behavior. Although I was a first-timer when it came to a final radiation treatment, Sue was not. "It's not unusual at all to feel the way you do. Most radiation patients experience a letdown." I needed and welcomed her compassionate support.

I was still crying when the department head entered the office for the routine appointment that followed the final treatment; and I told her of my unexpected feelings. She, too, was understanding and explained the void that was engulfing me. For almost a year, my life had been carefully scheduled. Under the care of a medical team, my life had revolved around my various medical appointments. Suddenly, my prescribed course of treatment was over—leaving an emotional void as well as a scheduling one.

As she went on to give me an overview of my follow-up care, I faced a new reality. I would not be able to close the breast cancer chapter in my life storybook today because the breast cancer chapter has an epilogue. It has an epilogue of follow-up care and appointments for a long time. The epilogue also includes ongoing physical, emotional, and relational healing and adjustments, as well as likely lifestyle changes. Although I felt deflated, I was grateful for her frankness.

Now, as I sit in the car reviewing her words, I sense a birthing within my void. Although I must face the reality that my yearning to return to normal pre-breast cancer life will never be fulfilled, I will not be leaving this radiation-therapy treatment center empty-handed. I can choose to fulfill the words of the Psalmist and leave carrying a bag of seeds. As I have gleaned valuable lessons and blessings during the breast cancer diagnosis and the treatment chapter in my life, I will likewise do so during my ongoing epilogue.

> **Dear God, I thank You for sustaining and blessing me through this chapter of my life. I now ask You to write the epilogue of my life from this day forward. I'm grateful for the promise in Psalm 126: Those who sow in tears shall reap with joyful shouting. Even as I weep, I can be assured that You will help me carry and sow my bag of seed so that I can, at the end of my epilogue, come with a shout of joy, bringing my sheaves with me. Amen.**

Compassion

And seeing the multitudes, He felt compassion for them, because they were distressed and downcast, like sheep without a shepherd. Then He said to His disciples, "The harvest is plentiful, but the workers are few. Therefore beseech the Lord of the harvest to send out workers into the harvest."

—Matthew 9:36-38

As I eagerly steered my car toward the lifted exit bar of the parking lot, I was vaguely aware of a faint door slam and a flicker of color to my distant left. Driving with the zeal of a bird heading for the open door of its cage, I continued on, anxious to leave behind me the radiation treatment center and its lingering connotations. It had been a month since my final treatment and the follow-up appointment day had gone well. Now I felt free and ready to move out and on.

But that bit of color caught in the corner of my eye snagged my attention and pulled my head to the left for a quick, curious look. Drawn in, my peek became a gaze as the source of the distraction captured my interest. The origin of the bit of color was a garment in motion, worn by a woman closing her car door and making her way across the lot to the radiation treatment center. The garment, however, was a stark contrast to the demeanor of the woman—stooped shoulders, labored movements, downcast expression.

I evidently was pausing too long at the exit bar. To my surprise, the woman turned her head my way and cast me a brief, furtive glance—one just long enough for her eyes to reveal her heavy burden of sadness, hopelessness, and pain. I was engulfed with a sense of compassion. Every fiber of my being was aching for her, longing to give her hope, wanting to somehow intervene in her behalf.

Out of the lot now and onto the busy street, I prayed that someone during the course of the woman's treatment would be a channel of hope and encouragement—that someone would see her need and respond with Christ-like compassion.

Christ-like compassion . . . As a Christian, my goal in life is to become more and more Christ-like. Is it possible that my breast cancer journey has allowed me to become more compassionate and therefore more Christ-like? If this startling possibility is true, than what do I do with this amazing compassion? Jesus himself has answered my question through his words, "Therefore beseech the Lord of the harvest to send out workers into His harvest."

His harvest . . . I know that the harvest refers to people—distressed and downcast people who are like sheep in need of a shepherd. I know what it is like to be distressed and downcast. I know Jesus, the Shepherd. I know His compassion, His salvation, His Lordship. Am I willing to be a channel of Jesus Christ's compassion? Am I willing to share the reality of the risen Christ, which I have experienced in the past and continue to experience now? Yes, with the help of my Shepherd, I will.

Dear Lord of the harvest, I'm grateful that You are the Shepherd of the distressed and downcast. Thank You for enabling me to become a woman of deeper compassion. Please help me to channel this compassion as a worker in Your harvest. Amen.

Help Wanted: Encourager

Therefore encourage one another, and build up one another.
—I Thessalonians 5:11

The pilot light on our gas fireplace had gone out several weeks ago. At the time, my husband made an unsuccessful attempt to correct the problem, but because it was early spring and we weren't using the fireplace, we forgot about its malfunction. An arctic cold front sweeping through Minnesota for one last farewell blast, however, jarred our memory and we longed for the cozy warmth of our fireplace.

"You better call the fireplace service center and tell them we need help fixing whatever's wrong," my husband advised as he left for work. "It's probably due to be serviced anyway," he said as he shivered in the doorway.

Following through, I provided the necessary information to the receptionist at the service center. "We'll have someone out between eleven and one o'clock on Thursday," she informed me. She paused and then ventured, "It will probably be Tim."

Thursday morning came, but the radio alarm sounded much too soon for me. I dozed off again and slept through my husband's grooming and dressing routines, breakfast, and our usual farewell rituals. The second time I woke up, I squinted at the clock and bolted out of bed. The waste-management truck was due any minute! I quickly cleaned up, dressed, and flew out the door. The truck had just left our driveway! With trash bags in tow, I chased on foot after the truck and thanked the driver profusely for responding to my plight.

That task accomplished, I went back into the house and collapsed on the kitchen chair. I felt as though I had just completed a full day of hard labor. "Will I ever get my energy back?" I wistfully wondered. I longed to be in full swing instead of dealing with this prolonged fatigue. I felt like an albatross had landed on my neck, was weighing me down, and refused to be shooed away.

Following my solitary breakfast and tidying up the kitchen, I relocated to the sunroom to write a few greeting cards and have my devotional time. As I was ending my prayer time, I remembered that the fireplace service man could be arriving soon. "And, Lord, please help me be a blessing to Tim," I concluded.

Within minutes, the doorbell rang and there was Tim. It was precisely eleven o'clock. With kind, sparkling eyes, he introduced himself, took off his shoes and placed them neatly by the door, and walked in to his work site.

Doing some writing a short distance away, I glanced up often to observe Tim at his work. What I saw filled me with surprise and appreciation. First, he laid out a canvas in front of the fireplace—clean side down—and carefully arranged his tools. He seemed to know exactly what to do and wasted no time in doing it. Removing the fireplace glass, he placed it on the canvas and thoroughly cleaned both sides—holding the glass up from time to time for inspection and further rubbing until it was smudge free. "This man enjoys his work and takes pride in doing it well," I thought to myself.

When he'd completed his servicing, Tim explained everything he'd done and offered to teach me how to correctly light the pilot. Grabbing a notepad and pen, I watched him and wrote down his instructions and tips as he patiently took me, step by step, through the procedure.

When we had finished, I couldn't resist asking, "Are you a Christian? You seem to radiate good will along with obvious competence in your trade. You emulate the ideal of a person who wants his work standard to reflect his beliefs. So . . . I'm wondering, are you a Christian?"

Tim blushed and replied, "Well, yes, I am. You're the second person who's asked me that question."

"Just before you rang the doorbell," I confessed, "I prayed that I'd be a blessing to you, but you've been a blessing and inspiration to me."

After we had briefly discussed our Christian beliefs, I mentioned that I was in the process of writing a devotional book for women experiencing breast cancer. "That's great!" Tim said. "Next year my wife will be a twenty-year breast cancer survivor."

As Tim prepared to leave, I told him that I had begun the day discouraged, but now was uplifted and eager to continue with my writing. He said that he was encouraged too. We shook hands and parted ways with a mutual, "God bless you."

The closed door behind me, I stood in our entry and pondered this unexpected source of strength and hope. I thanked God for His provision of help. I resumed my day, awed and revitalized by the wonder of God's intervention.

Dear God, it is beyond my understanding to grasp how You intervene in the mundane activities of everyday life. Thank You for the astounding ways You transcend our expectations to reveal Your caring and provision. Thank You for the blessing of encouraging and being encouraged, of building up and being built up. Following Your ways brings contentment and joy. Amen.

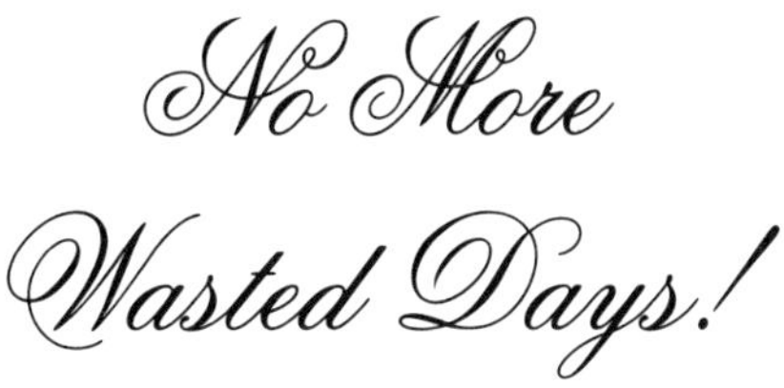

No More Wasted Days!

So teach us to number our days, that we may present to thee a heart of wisdom.

—Psalm 90:12 (NAS)

Teach us to number our days and recognize how few they are; help us to spend them as we should.

—Psalm 90:12 (LB)

"This is going to be one of those wasted days," I grumbled to myself midway through the morning. There had been a spring storm during the night, disrupting sleep for my husband and me. "Are you practicing keeping your eyes open?" Colin teased with our private joke as we fumbled around the kitchen getting breakfast to the table.

After we had exchanged parting waves, I considered going back to bed for another hour. However, I stubbed my toe on the leg of the bed frame and the pain jolted me into abrupt alertness. Sitting on the edge of the bed massaging my toe, I reviewed my current lot in life. Having recently completed seven weeks of radiation treatment, I still often felt fatigued—even after a full night's sleep. Now this day had barely begun and I was already feeling glum and contentious.

A flicker of black outside the bedroom window diverted my attention to the bird feeder on the deck. There, a loathsome crow was greedily devouring the fresh seed we'd put in the feeder to attract songbirds. Glad for something to vent my crabbiness on, I made a fist and pounded it on the window. My beady-eyed foe flew reluctantly to a nearby tree and scolded me with its blaring, abrasive "caw-caw."

"Well caw-caw to you too!" I spouted back. I was in no mood to be out-cawed this morning! It was 7:15 and I was already reduced to a cawing match with a crow. This was going to be a bad day.

Moving into the bathroom, I scowled at my reflection in the mirror. My eyes looked just as beady as that blasted crow's—except mine were framed in red. I debated putting on some makeup, at least something to conceal the blue bags under my eyes. Glowering into the mirror, I decided not to bother.

I morosely scrutinized the spring clothes recently brought out of storage. Perceiving everything in my wardrobe to be frumpy and blah, I selected garments as drab as I felt. The pants were snug. "How could my spring clothes possibly be snug?" I demanded. After all those weeks of no appetite or functioning taste buds during chemo, my pants are too tight? My fuming was followed by a wave of disappointment—I had allowed myself the silver-lining hope that I'd be down a size this spring. Well, so much for that fantasy.

Remembering that my husband had asked me to call about some trees, I went to his desk to find the telephone number. My futile search was interrupted by the ringing telephone. It was my husband, wondering what I had found out about the trees. "I haven't been able to find the phone number!" I testily retorted. "You should have given me the number before you left!" Grumbling under my breath, I called the tree nursery.

That out of the way, I sat down to have my daily quiet time of devotions, journaling, and prayer. I felt heavy-hearted after dumping my frustrations on my husband. He was likely to be struggling with fatigue too. Most of the clutter on his desk was mine. In fact, my stuff seemed to be cluttering the whole house. Our home had been neglected during the months of chemo and radiation treatments—and it showed.

The long list of to-do tasks looming before me distracted my mind as I read the devotionals. Flipping open my journal, I thought, "What should I write? Today is a wasted day?"

It was then that I read the Scripture reference printed across the bottom of the blank journal page. "So teach us to number our days, That we may present to Thee a heart of wisdom. Psalm 90:12."

Jarred out of my peevish mood, I read Psalm 90:12 in every translation I could find. Each translation revealed the same truth—wasted days are never God's plan.

I paused to consider how I would live this day if I knew that my number of remaining days were few. I certainly would not waste it out-cawing crows and snapping at my husband.

"I'm sorry," I prayed, "please forgive me and help me to value this day and live it wisely." I asked God to give me a second chance at this day and to see it with fresh eyes. Walking to the closet, I changed into something more comfortable and attractive. Next, I applied a touch of makeup. Feeling more civil already, I called my husband at work and passed on the information I'd gathered about the trees. I told him I was feeling better, and we had a brief, pleasant, mutually uplifting chat.

And then an amazing thought popped into my mind: "Write a devotional about the happenings of this day." We all get only one opportunity to live each day. We all have a limited number of days to live. We all would be wise to vow, "No more wasted days!"

Dear God, as I look back on my breast cancer experience, I realize it has forced me not to take life for granted. Thank You for allowing my breast cancer to bring me to a deeper awareness that my days on this earth are numbered. Whether my days are few or many, they are a gift from You. Please forgive me for having foolishly wasted days in the past. Help me to wisely live my remaining days. I do want to present to you a heart of wisdom. Please show me how. Amen.

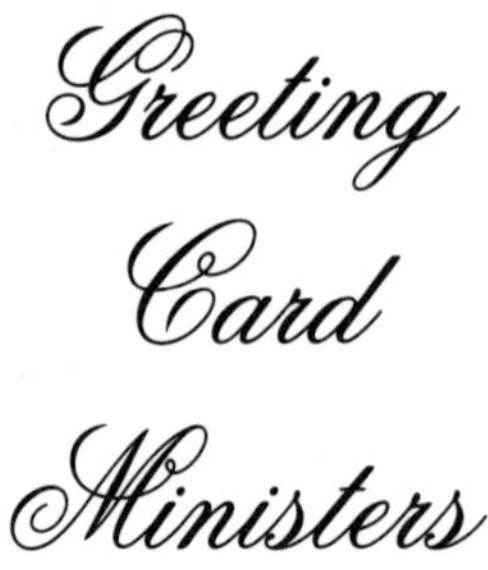

Greeting Card Ministers

We have different gifts, according to the grace given us . . . . If it is serving, let him serve . . . . If it is encouraging, let him encourage.

—Romans 12:6-8

There are many kinds of ministers, I've come to realize. Since childhood, I've known about the "official" ministers—those who are called and ordained to serve as clergy. I thank God for the generations of official ministers who have blessed so many lives, including mine.

During the course of my breast cancer treatment, however, I've come to recognize and appreciate another group of ministers. Their ministry is carried out behind the scenes, quietly and without fanfare, within the sanctuary of their homes. Their gift is delivered bearing a postage stamp and enclosed in an envelope sealed with caring and love. I call them greeting card ministers.

As the months of my treatment progressed, greeting cards and their senders took on a significance I had never before considered or imagined possible. Without exception, every greeting card I received blessed me. I displayed the cards where I could see them often. I enjoyed their beauty. I was inspired by the words they contained—the preprinted words as well as the words added by the sender.

I was often amazed that just the right kind of greeting card would arrive for my specific need. When laughter was the medicine I most needed, an outrageously hilarious card would arrive to tickle my funny bone. When I was longing for a touch of artistic expression, a creative card—handcrafted by pressing flowers, stamping, or mounting a photograph—would be delivered. When I felt spiritually dry, a card containing an appropriate Scripture reference would be in the mailbox. Every card was a gift in its own unique way. As my collection grew, I placed the cards in a wicker basket where I could choose one to reread and reflect upon as needed.

Gradually, it began to occur to me that certain people seemed to have a true ministry of serving and encouraging through greeting cards. For me, four particular women heeded God's call to be greeting card ministers during my breast cancer treatment: Shirley, Mary, Carol, and Laurie

Shirley is married to my husband's brother Bill. Cards from her are sometimes inspirational and at other times humorous, but they always include a note or letter updating me on what is happening with her and her family. I appreciate her including me in the loop of her life. I am grateful for the family God gave me when I married, and for this sister-in-law who helps me feel loved and valuable within this family. Shirley's ministry is motivated by caring.

Mary, also my sister-in-law, is married to my brother Mark. Mary is a woman of many moods, from A to Z—angelic to zany. Her cards convey messages for the mood of the day and bring a joke, a lovely illustration, a poem, or a passage to ponder. With so many moods and so many cards to choose from, how does she always make the ideal choice? I asked her once. Mary said, "Oh, I don't know . . . I just knew that card was for you." I believe that the Holy Spirit knows my need and guides Mary's selection.

Carol, a sister, is three years younger than I am. Growing up, we shared the same room, but our personalities and interests seemed so different that I sometimes wondered if we would ever be truly close. Then, as young adults, we embarked on similar faith journeys and have since grown very intimate in our mutual faith in Jesus.

Some of the qualities I especially love and admire in Carol are expressed in these cliches: "What you see is what you get"; and "She wears her heart on her sleeve." There are no false pretenses with Carol. When she feels deeply, she freely expresses her sentiments with her emotions and words. That genuineness anoints the cards she sends to me. As I hold each card, I sense her unbridled love ministering, encouraging, and binding us ever closer.

Laurie is my "younger woman" friend. Our paths first crossed years ago when I was a young married mom and she was a high school girl. We both attended a Saturday evening Bible study-worship-prayer group that merged our hearts and spirits.

Laurie delights in life and new ventures. As her career carries her to various cities, she sends a picture postcard—her latest news hugging the margins of the message side. While I remain in the healing comfort of my home, Laurie's picture postcards reach across the miles, inviting me to join vicariously in her travels and new experiences.

Today I could use a greeting card minister! It's that time of year in the Minnesota theater of seasons when spring makes her reentrance on center stage. She teases with her brief flirtations of warmth and sunshine, only to turn her back and prance away—leaving dreary old winter to perform an encore again and again. March entered like a lion this spring and, for the most part, continues to roar a chilly wind—forcing equally dreary me to bundle up just to retrieve the mail from the box.

I find mostly junk mail—except for a greeting card from Laurie! Hurrying back to the house, I feel that my day is already brightened. This time Laurie has sent, not a picture postcard, but a card crafted by her photographer aunt. A smile transforms my face as I bask in the card's beauty and underlying message. Two tulips—one red and one yellow—are shown blooming through a blanket of snow.

God has again used one of his greeting card ministers to deliver a message. The certain hope of springtime is here, not only for nature, but also for me. I am emerging from my long winter of cancer treatment-induced dormancy, and I will bloom again—just as surely as the tulips on the card before me. I have been ministered to. I am encouraged.

Dear Caller to ministry, according to Your grace, You give your children many different kinds of gifts. It is You who prompts and calls us to diverse ministries. Thank You for those who heed Your call to minister and to encourage needy hearts and spirits through greeting cards. I ask You to bless and anoint them in their mission. Amen.

Martha or Mary?

But the Lord answered and said to her, "Martha, Martha, you are worried and bothered about so many things; but only a few things are necessary, really only one, for Mary has chosen the good part, which shall not be taken away from her."

—Luke 10:41,42

"Sharon, Sharon, you are worried and bothered about so many things," became, several years ago, a caution I repeated to myself often. I had begun the custom of spending part of a January day alone with God. With Bible, prayer journal, and pen in hand, I'd ask God to guide me in writing a special prayer for my husband, for each of our children, and for myself. These were the prayers I would include during my daily prayer time throughout the new year.

One particular year, the Martha and Mary Scripture reference came clearly to my mind as I waited for God to guide me in writing the foundational prayer for myself. As I looked up and read the passage in Luke 10:38-42, I wondered, "Am I a Martha or a Mary?" God seemed to impress upon my spirit the need for me to grow away from my Martha tendencies and toward Mary's priority. Committing the Scripture to God as the basis for my prayer, I asked Him to help in my transformation process.

An unusual occurrence began to happen on a regular basis. Whenever my mind and body would be gripped by anxiety, the words, "Sharon, Sharon, you are worried and bothered about so many things," would clearly come to my mind. The words would caution me to halt my harried pace and take a time-out with God. I would visualize myself temporarily setting aside all my Martha responsibilities and quietly, expectantly, sitting by Mary at the feet of Jesus. Then, as I was still before Jesus, God would calm me and help me put my responsibilities and tasks into perspective. God would help me align my priorities with His will for my life.

It took the whole year of reflecting, praying, being receptive to inner healing, and responding in many practical ways to the Martha and Mary passage for me to progress in my transformation process. Although a different passage and prayer came forth the next year, I've continued to be gradually changed by the relevance of Jesus' loving, guiding words to Martha—and to me.

* * *

This morning, in the midst of my flurry of thoughts and plans, a quiet whisper found its way to my mind and spirit: "Sharon, Sharon, you are worried and bothered about so many things."

"Where did that come from? And why?" I wondered. Then I knew where and why. God, in His gentle, sure care, knew that I was allowing my priorities to become skewed again.

Since my breast cancer diagnosis, I've become much less Martha-like and much more Mary-like. I simply didn't have the stamina to keep up with the Martha in me. In channeling time and energy toward healing and restored health, I identified more and more with Mary. Being still and receptive to my Lord's presence and His involvement in my life is so satisfying that I yearn for an ever-deepening relationship with Him. I wanted to remain intimate with Him and attuned to His guidance.

During my breast cancer experience, I discovered that there are benefits to having fewer expectations placed upon me: I'd been given permission—so to speak—to step off the merry-go-round of life-as-usual. I'd been allowed the luxury of stillness, rest, and healing.

I wanted the valuable lessons I've learned to bear the fruit of an ongoing healthier, more balanced lifestyle.

Lately, with my last radiation treatment behind me, my mind is often racing—eager to catch up with the myriad tasks neglected during my long course of treatment. My body, however, is uncooperative. Like mismatched dance partners, my mind wants to hurry to the middle of the floor and jitterbug, while my wallflower body is content to rest on the sidelines.

So, who am I now? A Martha or a Mary? Neither, I conclude. I am a Sharon, with the best and the worst of both Martha and Mary. I, like Martha and Mary, am continually in need of Jesus' companionship and guidance.

Dear Lord, I come to You with my Martha tendencies to become so worried and bothered about the responsibilities and tasks of life that I neglect what's most important. I thank You for my season of becoming more like Mary. Please help me to be the woman You desire me to be. Amen.

Looking Back, Looking Forward

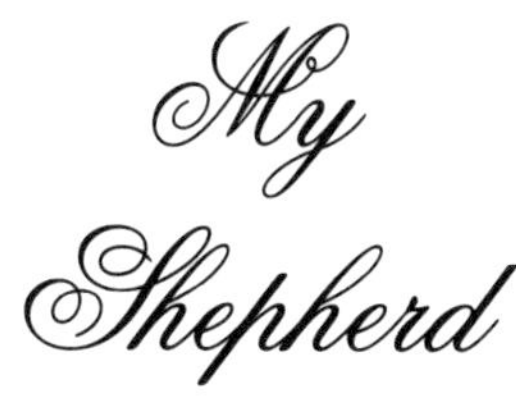

My Shepherd

The Lord is my shepherd, I shall not want.

—Psalm 23:1

The stained-glass window in the church sanctuary depicting Jesus as a shepherd once again serves as my teacher. Over and over through the years, my attention has wandered away from the church service and lingered on the scene that has graced the south wall of the sanctuary since 1909. Always the same, yet ever-changing with the nuances of the sun's rays.

The Good Shepherd image was in my life long before I actually knew or had a relationship with the Shepherd of shepherds. I recall seeing it as a framed print, a ceramic plaque, a sketch on a bookmark, and in many other forms and places.

It took on new meaning six years prior to my breast cancer diagnosis when I became the founding director of the Shepherd's Center, an interdenominational service agency by and for senior adults. Founding the first Shepherd's Center in the state was a calling that I felt I could answer only through my total dependence on the Shepherd.

During the year of establishing the center, I came often to church to sit in the pew closest to the feet of the Shepherd. Gazing up at the Shepherd, I prayed for guidance step by step, month by month.

Most days I felt like the helpless little lamb cradled in the Shepherd's arms. I sensed the calling to found Shepherd's

Center was beyond my personality, training, and abilities. I needed the passion, wisdom, strength, and insights of the Great Shepherd to move on to each new phase.

As the months progressed, prayers were answered and it became clear to me and to others that God was guiding and blessing the development of Shepherd's Center. Accolades were coming my way and I didn't feel the desperate need to go to the pew by the stained-glass window to pray.

Thankfully, I heeded the nudge of the Holy Spirit to go anyway. God directed my eyes, not to the helpless lamb in the arms of Jesus, but rather to the lead sheep. This sheep appeared mature, strong, and healthy—a leader prepared to launch off on its own. But . . . the eyes of the lead sheep were not turned toward some path heading into the distance; rather they were fixed on the eyes of the Shepherd. The body of the lead sheep remained close to the Shepherd, touching the folds of His garment.

God used the image to teach me that even when I am feeling strong, healthy, mature, bold, and confident, it is important to stay close to Him for protection and guidance. Launching out on my own places me in danger of undue inflating of my ego, swayed priorities, misguided direction, and other obstacles that could hinder or mar His best.

My eyes have looked at the Good Shepherd window so often over the years since then that I no longer need to go to the church to recall the image. My mind's eye can now visualize the Shepherd and the sheep anytime, anywhere.

What lesson is the Good Shepherd teaching me today? For the past months of treatment and healing, I have related most often to the lamb being carried in the Shepherd's arms. Now that my course of treatment is over, I am regaining strength and stamina. I am allowing my thoughts to venture beyond yesterday and today and to move into the future.

As I dream of my future with eagerness and confidence, I am being reminded to keep my eyes fixed on the Shepherd and to walk close beside Him, secure in the folds of His garment. I need the unchanging Shepherd each moment of my ever-changing life.

Dear Shepherd, sometimes I feel like a helpless little lamb, precious and safe in Your strong, sure arms. At other times, I feel my own strength and confidence urging me to charge out into the world ahead of You. Help me to remember to remain so close that my gaze is always on You, my will enfolded in Your touch. Only then will I not stray from Your best for me. Amen.

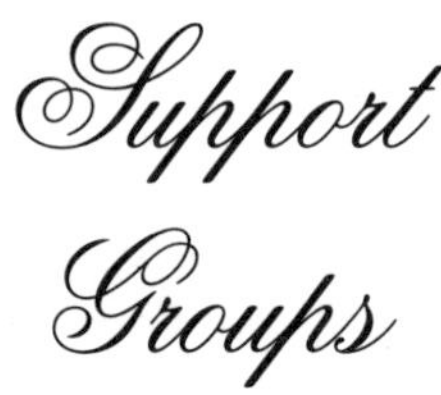

Let no unwholesome word proceed from your mouth, but only such a word as is good for edification according to the need of the moment, that it may give grace to those that hear.

—Ephesians 4:29

I hadn't planned to attend multiple support groups, but the opportunity seemed to naturally evolve over the course of my treatment. I attended three breast cancer support groups for a varying number of sessions. In so doing, I was struck by the distinct flavor of each group—and the nature and power of the words that were spoken at each.

The first group I attended met in the small city that I drove to for clinic appointments with my primary physician, my surgeon, and my oncologist. The cofacilitators, both breast cancer survivors, were zealous in their commitment to supporting women experiencing breast cancer. Each time I attended, fifteen to twenty women were seated around the large conference table. It was a well-established group.

Its focus was sharing information, offering support, and sponsoring an occasional special event. The tone was welcoming and warm and exuded the freedom to ask dumb questions and express emotions, whatever they might be. Although this was not a group based on a particular religious faith, the value of faith, prayer, and other sources of spiritual strength such as

Scripture, quotes, poems, and stories were readily shared with all the members.

Several of the women in the group were long-term survivors, yet continued to attend so they could be ongoing givers and receivers of encouragement. It was clear that the facilitators and the regulars cared about one another—and about me, the newcomer. Mouths were guarded, not to inhibit speaking candidly, but to guard against words that would discourage, fuel fear, or injure rather than aid. The group was truly a service and a blessing.

The second support group I attended was at a large metropolitan hospital. Two women, both part of the medical staff at the hospital, led this group of twenty women representing a wide range of ethnic, educational, and socioeconomic backgrounds. As in the first group I attended, the facilitators began by inviting each woman to introduce herself and share a bit about her breast cancer experience. Again, as in the first group, there was the freedom to express thoughts and emotions.

The tone of this group, however, was decidedly different than the first I'd attended. I was taken aback by the voiced anger, criticism, bitterness, and sarcasm. Negative experiences with treatment, medical staff, and prostheses escalated into a "Who can top this?" sharing of stories. One first-timer nervously shared that she would begin chemotherapy the next week. Instead of being supported, the woman was besieged with tales of woe. Noting the woman's growing anxiety level, I injected that my experience had been quite bearable. Dismissed as an oddity, I had to wait until the mid-session break to privately offer the encouragement omitted by the "support" group.

Was this a typical session—this runaway venting with no guidance or intervention by the facilitators or group members? I don't know. It certainly is possible that those who vented less than positive emotions and experiences found the group therapeutic. Although I continued to receive notices of the group meetings, I never was able to motivate myself to return. Perhaps it was a supportive group for others, but it wasn't a good fit for me.

Later, the flyer headline, "Faith-Based Breast Cancer Support Group" caught my attention. Noting that the first meeting was just days away and that the church location was within a reasonable distance, I decided to attend. The woman convening the group was outgoing and vivacious—a breast cancer survivor and member of the host church. She said this was a volunteer ministry she was eager to begin.

Several of those attending the group were not being treated for breast cancer. One young woman came because her mother was dying of breast cancer several states and thousands of miles away. She was in tears, grieving her inability to be with her mother during these final weeks. An elderly man was there with his wife, adult daughter, and granddaughter. He was a hospice patient, near the end of his battle with terminal cancer.

The group participants shared words of their experience, compassion, and prayer. The only uneasiness I perceived was in the facilitator. With all respect to her commendable motives, generous and loving heart, and capable leadership, she was uncomfortable with silence and rushed in to speak for group members. There is a time when being silent is the best way to honor the admonition, "Set a guard, O Lord, over my mouth; keep watch over the door of my lips."

Three breast cancer support groups. Three unique gatherings of God's loved ones. There were mouths that were guarded and mouths that were unguarded. There were mouths that spoke to offer encouragement, despair, compassion, bitterness, fear, faith, love, anger, defeat, and hope. There were mouths that spoke too much, too little, not at all. There were lips that smiled, lips that quivered, lips that channeled tiny rivulets of tears.

What did I learn from my breast cancer support groups? I learned that every such group is unique. I learned that these groups vary in the carrying out of their intended mission to assist and strengthen. I learned that it behooves me and others to inquire about the group's facilitators, participants, goals, and tone. I learned that God can and does bless through support groups. If a group isn't a blessing, another group can be found that is. An appropriate support group is a treasure worth seeking.

> **Dear Triune God, every encounter is an opportunity to support and be supported. I ask You to set a guard over my mouth and keep watch over the door of my lips as I live out my days with others who need and are needed. Thank you, God, Jesus Christ, and Holy Spirit, for being my Divine Support Group. Amen.**

Friends

"Greater love has no one than this, that one lay down his life for his friends."

—John 15:13

Looking back over the course of my breast cancer treatment, I realize that my understanding of friendship has taken on a deeper and broader dimension. During my encounter with breast cancer, the water through which I viewed friendship became muddied before it became clear.

There were the surprises of acquaintances who seemed to come out of the woodwork to extend the hand of friendship. There were those with whom I had forged friendships years ago, with whom cancer served as a catalyst to reconnect in a closer bond than ever. There were strangers who, while sharing my journey for a time, became new friends.

Finally, there were those friends who seemed to disappear just when I needed them most. I didn't know what to feel about these fair-weather friends. Surprise? Chagrin? Loss? It was while puzzling over this group of friends that I was forced to come to God with a teachable heart, ask why, and grow through His answer.

* * *

Friends—Lars, as one of my husband's university housemates was affectionately known, became my friend as the three of us shared meals, kitchen duties, and spiritual growth at one of the campus ministry centers. As we eventually earned degrees and pursued our respective career paths, Lars settled in another state, and our friendship was soon relegated to the confines of an annual Christmas letter exchange.

Thirty-five years later, in my husband's and my time of need, Lars came once again to the forefront of our friendships and became a channel through whom God answered a very significant prayer. Lars was the practicing and teaching surgeon at the university hospital to whom I referred in the devotional, "Second Opinion—Second Surgery." He rallied to our rescue like a knight in shining armor—or in his case, a surgeon in shining scrubs—to offer not only his medical expertise and contacts, but also genuine caring, and the emotional and prayer support of a true friend.

* * *

Friends—Ruth and I share a relationship that can be likened to a friendship bracelet with an ever-increasing number of links. The first link, transition, came when we both left small-town schools in rural communities and entered the University of Minnesota as incoming freshmen. The second link followed when, as college students, we shared the same dormitory, major, classes, professors, sorority, and graduation ceremony.

Our adventures as vagabonds was the third link, acquired the summer following our graduation, as Ruth, another young woman, and I—clutching our meager financial resources and possessions—boarded a Youth Hostel airplane and took flight for Europe. Following our incredible summer abroad, we returned to Minnesota and our fourth link, teaching careers. Soon we added the fifth link, marriage, and the sixth, motherhood. Although we lived scarcely an hour's drive apart, our seventh link, busy lives, kept our friendship at a distance—maintained by annual holiday correspondence and an occasional get-together.

Ruth and I never anticipated that we would some day add—albeit not of our own choosing—an eighth link to our friendship bracelet as breast cancer patients. Ruth's diagnosis and treatment followed a year behind mine and served as an impetus for us to revitalize our relationship. With each contact made, our friendship bond deepened as I supported Ruth through her course of treatment and she supported me in my writing of devotionals for women experiencing breast cancer.

❋ ❋ ❋

Friends—During the course of my chemotherapy and radiation treatments, my husband and I were in our third of a five-year living situation during which we rented out our rural farm home during the school term so that we could live in a suburban townhouse near Colin's school job. The primary reason for our unusual living arrangement was to allow Colin's back, injured while working on the farm and aggravated by the two-hour-a-day commute, to heal.

Returning to our townhouse following my summer of diagnosis and surgeries, Colin and I learned that our next-door neighbor, Pam, would be home on medical leave for the school term. In our mutual concern for each other's well-being, Pam and I began a routine of almost daily check-in calls. When weather permitted, we opted for a walk instead of a phone call. By the end of the school term in June, we had developed a close, enduring friendship. We remain in awe of how God brought us together as neighbors during our parallel season of treatment and healing—of how God works in mysterious ways, His wonders to perform.

❋ ❋ ❋

Friends—"What about my fair-weather friends?" I wondered more and more as the weeks, then months of my course of treatment progressed with little or no contact from a few people whom I had perceived to be close friends. Bewildered, I asked myself, "Have I done something to distance our friendship? Has it been a one-sided friendship all along?" Eventually, I took my frustration and hurt to God and asked, "What's going on here?"

God's answer was quite unexpected. He drew my attention to my hand with a finger pointing in accusation toward my fair-weather friends. Prompted to study my hand, I noted that three of my fingers were pointing back at me. God brought to my mind a number of times when friends of mine had been experiencing difficult times. As He gently but clearly brought to my mind the responses I had made, I realized that I had failed as a friend many times. "How could I have let down my friends during their time of need?" I asked myself.

As I revisited those times when I had been a negligent friend, I realized that sometimes I had felt too inadequate, too awkward, or too fearful to make a contact or provide support. Other times I had harbored noble intentions but, swept up in the seemingly urgent business of my life, I had put off the important contact gesture until it was embarrassingly tardy or altogether too late. The remorse I felt as I acknowledged my own shortcomings as a friend overshadowed the disappointment I was feeling toward my friends who, like me, are only human.

Glancing again at my hand with one finger pointing in accusation and three fingers bent under pointing back at me, I knew it was time to change its position. I lifted my open hand to God, as I prayed, "Forgive me my trespasses as I forgive those who trespass against me."

Friends—When with His disciples, Jesus spoke of a love so great that one is willing to lay down his life for his friends. Jesus practiced what He preached. My muddy-water understanding of friendship is now clearer. All friends are gifts from God—to be loved as Jesus loves.

Dear Jesus, thank You for the gift of friends—past, present, and future. I yearn for a deeper relationship with You, my Divine Friend, so that I may develop a greater, more sacrificial love for my friends. Please help me become the friend You desire me to be. Amen.

Priorities Examined

"But seek first His kingdom and His righteousness; and all these things shall be added to you."

—Matthew 6:33

The scene played before my closed eyes like a theatrical production. The setting was Tokyo, Japan, in 1984. My husband, our children, and I were short-term missionaries serving as parents for the girls' dormitory at a Christian boarding school. Most of our fifteen dorm daughters were the children of career missionaries.

It seemed like a responsibility that continued day and night—every day. I certainly knew why God doesn't give most parents a total of eighteen children. And in this case, fifteen of them were teenaged girls from several different countries!

Despite our huge family, the culture shock, and the challenge of financing our mission work, we received many extraordinary blessings during our two-year stint of service. I, however, was often too overwhelmed by my hour-to-hour, day-to-day responsibilities to notice.

One day, Amy, one of our eleventh-grade dorm daughters, bounced into the living room-lounge after school. "Where does she get her energy?" I thought feeling a hint of irritation and self-pity. While she had spent the day in school, I had completed my daily routine of checking the girls' rooms. Then I'd traveled by train to another section of Tokyo to teach English conversation and Bible to my "Wednesday group" of Japanese women, stopped on the way back to buy groceries, and now was preparing the oyatsu (snack) to be served during the evening gathering for family devotions. I was exhausted.

Oblivious to my state of mind, Amy plunked herself near me and with exuberance shared her pearl of news: "Mother Teresa is in Tokyo and has invited a small group of missionary kids to an audience with her on Friday. I've been selected to go! I asked if you could be one of the adult chaperones. Isn't this amazing?"

Without thinking, without prayer, I followed only the instincts of my weary mood and replied, "Sorry, Amy. I have so much I have to do Friday, I won't possibly be able to get away for such a big chunk of the day."

Amy's deflated smile and countenance contradicted her attempt to retain a measure of cheerfulness as she expressed her assurance that certainly another adult could be found to take my place.

Mistaken decisions, birthed from skewed priories, breed regret that matures over a lifetime of revisiting the scenes of yesteryear. In this case I have long forgotten what the duties were that loomed in such magnitude, such significance, with such unyielding deadlines as to warrant my willingness to be robbed of a once-in-a-lifetime opportunity. Writing a newsletter article? Doing the laundry? Cleaning the bathroom? Whatever it was, the outcome blares in exemplification of the old adage of "the tyranny of the urgent over the important." There was no second chance to have a private audience with Mother Teresa before she died.

Because we have a God of second chances, however, my regret over the mistaken decision has served as an impetus to encounter Mother Teresa in other ways. I have taken the time to glean from the documentary film of her life, as well as from several television and printed interviews, the profound wisdom she offered.

One of the benefits of breast cancer is that it forces an examination of one's life. In so doing, there is the opportunity to reminisce, view priorities from a new vantage point, and rethink the future. Whether this chance at life is a first, second, third, or beyond, it is the gift of a pivotal juncture to examine priorities and birth a future free of regrets.

Dear God, I'm grateful for Your mercy, grace, and wisdom. In Your mercy, please forgive my decisions that have missed the mark of Your best for me. In Your grace, allow my breast cancer experience to open my eyes to mistaken priorities in my past. In Your wisdom, guide my priorities for the remainder of my life. Amen.

Lessons from the Journey

Therefore, since we are justified by faith, we have peace with God through our Lord Jesus Christ. Through him we have obtained access to this grace in which we stand, and we rejoice in our hope of sharing the glory of God. More than that, we rejoice in our suffering, knowing that suffering produces endurance, and endurance produces character, and character produces hope, and hope does not disappoint us, because God's love has been poured into our hearts through the Holy Spirit which has been given to us.

—Romans 5:1-5 (RSV)

Looking back over my breast cancer journey, I realize that I've learned many lessons along the way. In fact, I've gleaned such valuable teachings applicable to life—whether touched by cancer or not—that I long to share some of them with others. "But which lessons?" I ask myself, because I realize that I have learned many—and I want to share them all.

The answer to my question came when I read Romans 5:1-5. The lessons I found in that passage to share? Suffering, endurance, character, and hope.

Suffering. The mere mention of the word makes us shudder. If someone were to announce, "Today I am here to offer you endurance, character, and hope. All you have to do is line up for suffering," I wonder how many people would rush forward to step in line?

I find it thought-provoking that Scripture associates suffering with the positives of endurance, character, and hope. How unlike our human and cultural way of thinking in which suffering is associated with negatives—pain, loss, tears, anguish. Let's admit it—most of us want to always feel comfortable and happy.

We tend to link suffering with bad news—a relationship changing for the worse; the death of someone dear; loneliness; a crisis related to health, job, or finances; or any of a myriad of struggles. No one likes to receive news that suffering will be part of the package. The day I was given the bad news of my cancer diagnosis, I also received another message: Whether of my choosing or not, I was stepping into the line for suffering.

Shortly after my diagnosis, I joined a busload of women from southeast Minnesota and attended the Women of Faith conference in Minneapolis. One of the speakers, Sheila Walsh, summarized the suffering experience of those awaiting the results of life-altering medical tests with these words: "Whether you get the news you are most hoping for or the news you most dread, God can be trusted equally either way."

As my year of treatment for breast cancer progressed, I realized I could trust God to be with me through the best days and the worst days. Thinking back, I realize my richest lessons were learned during my most difficult days, the days I endured the most suffering.

Endurance is defined as the capacity to keep going or put up with pain or hardship for a long time. I'd thought I already had the quality of endurance. After all, I sometimes teased my husband, I had been married to him for over thirty-three years! Besides that, my ethnic heritage is predominantly Finnish. The Finns are known for their "sisu," a Finnish word that translates to "true grit" or endurance.

More important, however, I had a history of knowing and trusting Jesus as my Savior and Lord, and I sensed I was "riding on a wave of prayer." I fully expected to ride on top of that wave every day—to outride fear and depression all of the time. Praise to God and thanks to those who hung in with me through prayer for the long haul, I was able to ride that wave during most of my journey—but certainly not for 100 percent of it.

There were days when I was so sick and tired of feeling sick and tired that I wanted to throw every cancer-related thing I owned into the trash and haul it out to the curb. I was also tempted to place the recycling bin alongside the trash barrel, climb inside, and hope a merciful waste management worker would recycle me into a healthy woman.

On other days, despite my faith and my support, I struggled with anxiety, fear, sadness, and other emotions I'm not sure I can even name. I needed to believe that my marathon breast cancer race wasn't a total waste of my life. I needed the validation that I found in Romans 5, verse 4: "and endurance produces character."

Character. I know now that I am not the same person I was before my breast cancer diagnosis. There's been a pruning of sorts so that new character growth could emerge.

- My down days forced me to share my needs with others. In doing so, I found my admission of perceived shortcomings and concerns often freed people to in turn share their struggles with me. As we supported each other and prayed, we were drawn closer to each other and to God.
- I've become a more empathetic and compassionate person toward others who are suffering and enduring.
- I've become a more grateful person—thankful for the abundant blessings that are mine to treasure.

- I no longer take time for granted, but have learned to value it highly. For almost a year I was nudged off the merry-go-round of life and adjusted my schedule to accommodate my medical treatment and healing needs. I was given a gift of time to experience in fresh new ways God's tenderness toward me as His beloved child, to think and pray deeply, and to be available to people who needed a listening ear, a word of encouragement, prayer—and even an offering of hope.

Hope. Romans 5, verse 4 continues, "and character produces hope, and hope does not disappoint us, because God's love has been poured into our hearts through the Holy Spirit that has been given to us." What do I hope, now that I have suffered, endured, and further developed my character?

Among other things, I hope cancer will never recur in my body. I hope I can live a long healthy life and be an influence for Christ to my children's children as my mother and mother-in-law have been for my children. But I have come to realize it is not the number of days in our life that matters so much as it is how we live the days we have.

We don't need to live our days clouded by hope-corroding fear of any situation or circumstance; 1 John 4:18 tells us "there is no fear in love because perfect love casts out all fear." I have found through my suffering, endurance, and character-building that the hope I have in God's love is indeed more powerful than my deepest fears. That is the hope I carry with me as I continue my life journey.

Dear God, I'm thankful for the peace I am able to have through our Lord Jesus Christ, and for the grace in which I stand. Thank You for the lessons of suffering, endurance, character, and hope I have learned during my breast cancer journey. I rejoice in my hope of sharing Your glory. Amen.

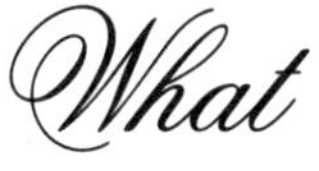

What is Beauty?

Charm is deceitful and beauty is vain, but a woman who fears the Lord, she will be praised.

—*Proverbs 31:30*

And let not your adornment be merely external . . . but let it be the hidden person of the heart, with the imperishable quality of a gentle and quiet spirit, which is precious in the sight of God.

—*1 Peter 3:3,4*

And in Him, you have been made complete.

—*Colossians 2:10*

"What is beauty?" is a question breast cancer forces a woman to ask anew. It is a question that deserves an insightful and truthful answer.

Breast cancer, I've come to realize, is a perpetrator that never invades alone. It always brings along its gang of cronies, each with its own potential to assault and diminish.

The crony that attacks self-image shows no mercy as it aims for the core of a woman's sense of femininity and wholeness. "You are unattractive. You are scarred. You aren't even a whole woman any more," taunts the self-image-destroying bully. This crony of breast cancer is one whose bluff must be confronted and defeated through God's victorious truth. But what is the truth about beauty?

During my childhood, subtle messages about beauty came through my favorite storybooks. Cinderella was beautiful; her ugly stepsisters were not. Snow White and Sleeping Beauty were beautiful. The ugly duckling was teased and excluded until after it was transformed into a beautiful swan. Physical beauty, I concluded by preadolescence, was the gateway to acceptance, attracting a handsome prince, and living happily ever after.

I first read Proverbs 31—sometimes referred to as the "worthy woman" passage—during my teenage years. This Scripture passage irked me—especially verse 30. It convinced me that God was totally out of touch with what it was like to be a blossoming young woman. Observing that most of the popular girls in my high school were attractive, my desire was to be charming and beautiful, despite a degree of fear that the Lord would someday judge me for rejecting the supposed wisdom of Proverbs 31:30.

Years later, I bought my first study Bible and was pleased to read in a footnote that "fear of the Lord" means loving reverence for God that includes a desire to release oneself to His Lordship and His word. "Lord," I prayed, "Even though I still want to be as attractive as possible, please help me become the woman You created me to be."

As time went on, I began to recognize that, indeed, charm can be deceitful and beauty can be vain. I became acquainted with several women who were beautiful, but were often self-centered, shallow, and insecure in their skin-deep perception of worth. I pondered, "When physical attractiveness begins to fade, as it inevitably does, these women may be forced to ask, 'Who am I aside from my beauty?'"

What is beauty? I became increasingly aware of the ability of inner beauty to radiate beyond the confines of natural attractiveness or cosmetic enhancement. I remembered the Old Testament account of God's words as He sent Samuel to chose a king from among the sons of Jesse: "Do not look at his appearance or at the height of his stature . . . for God sees not as man sees, but the Lord looks at the heart" (1 Samuel 16:7).

Jesus, as prophesied by Isaiah, would not be esteemed for being handsome, but rather he would have "no stately form or majesty that we should look upon Him, nor appearance that we should be attracted to Him" (Isaiah 53:2).

My daughter Krissy taught me a lesson about beauty that reinforces Scripture's teachings. When she began a new term as an elementary school student, Krissy often raved about her beautiful teacher. By the time fall parent-teacher conferences arrived, I was prepared to meet a beauty queen.

Instead, the teacher's physical appearance was quite plain. Within minutes into the conference, however, I too viewed the teacher as an extraordinarily beautiful woman. The sparkle that gleamed in her eyes and her glowing countenance of love for her students transcended physical features.

Perhaps the most striking contrast between outer and inner beauty was evident to me as I viewed the documentary movie of Mother Teresa's life. After following the compassionate nun as she touched and ministered to the unlovliest of the unlovely and the poorest of the poor, the movie culminated with Mother Teresa receiving the Nobel Peace Prize.

The other women present at the award ceremony were beautifully coifed, groomed, and dressed. When Mother Teresa entered the ceremony—simply adorned in her customary blue-trimmed white sari, her inner spiritual beauty illuminated the room and the outward beauty of the other women paled in comparison.

What is beauty? I found further insight in this quote from *The Mystery of God's Will,* by Charles R. Swindoll: "God will not look you over for medals, degrees, or diplomas, but for scars." Neither will God, I believe, look us over for beauty-queen tiaras, but for our scars and what we did about them. After all, the storybooks that formed my perception of beauty during my childhood days were just that—stories in a book. In our real world, it is a rare or nonexistent woman who makes it through life without being scarred—physically, emotionally, or spiritually.

Our scars can either mar or enhance our beauty. In reality, our scars, rather than our genetics, may give us the greater choice in determining our beauty. Although our scars in themselves may not be beautiful, they carry the potential to bring about an inner beauty that cannot be lost through a surgeon's knife, nor fade with age, nor establish the boundaries of womanhood, nor define worth.

What determines whether our scars rob or enhance our beauty? I believe the answer lies in Scripture and in our willingness to believe its truth. The answer lies in the example of the woman in Proverbs 31:30 "who fears [lovingly reveres] the Lord, she shall be praised." The answer lies in the example of Jesus' scars on His scourged body, the scars on His hands and feet—the scars that represent His dying on the cross and being raised again so that we may have an abundant life, an eternal life. Because of what Jesus did with His scars, every woman is without blemish, beautiful to Him, complete in Him.

Dear Lord, thank You for helping me grow deeper in my understanding of beauty, scars, and wholeness. You know my scars—those that are visible to others, those that I see, and those that You alone are aware of. I give my scars to You—to heal and to use to enhance my beauty. I thank You for the scars You endured in Your great love for me. Help me know that I am a beautiful and complete woman because of You. Amen.

Changed Relationships

And we know that God causes all things to work together for good to those who love God, to those who are called according to His purpose.
—Romans 8:28

I suppose breast cancer impacted many of my relationships in some way, but three especially stand out. My relationships with my mother, with my husband, and with God changed in very positive ways because of my breast cancer experience.

Whether the strong work ethic was a reflection of the times, the rural and ethnic character of the community, the dynamics of my family, or all three, I don't know. I do know I perceived work to reign paramount during my childhood and teenage years.

Unbeknownst to anyone but God, I yearned to spend time with my mother that didn't revolve around work. Work seemed to be never-ending and shaped much of my relationship with my mother. Although Mom and I loved and respected each other, I longed for us to make fun memories together that had nothing to do with work.

My breast cancer, especially the five months of chemotherapy, was hard on Mom. She expressed her own longing—to help in whatever way she could. Transportation arrangements were made through the assistance of relatives and friends, and Mom would come to stay for a few days at a time. "Be sure you make a list of 'jobbies' for me to do," Mom reminded me prior to each visit.

During her first trip, I gave her the job of cleaning a drawer in the kitchen. As I rested and watched her at work, my heart's desire found its voice: "Mom, what I really want and need most is for us to do something fun together." What followed was the first of many little mother-daughter adventures. Our outings were so deeply satisfying for both of us, they are continuing even though my course of treatment is now over.

I have never loved, treasured, and enjoyed my mother as much as I do now. Not everything that accompanies breast cancer is a foe. Sometimes even breast cancer can be used by God to make secret dreams come true.

* * *

I still break into the smile of a young woman in love when I think about one particular morning. My course of treatment for breast cancer was behind me, and I was gradually regaining stamina. That day, I was sitting in our sunroom. There was no sun shining in the room, however, and I was feeling as gloomy as the overcast sky. Taking my cue from the grey clouds, I was dolefully reading my daily devotional book.

Just as I was lifting my hand to turn a page, the sun broke through the clouds—its rays beaming directly on my diamond engagement ring. Although the ring had been on my hand for thirty-three years, I had never before seen such a spectrum of vibrant colors radiating from the diamond.

Caught up in the wonder of the moment, I rotated my hand slightly, and delighted in the resulting show of dancing colors. As the light-and-color display prompted me to note the many facets of my diamond ring, it also beckoned me to consider the many facets of my marriage. Each facet seemed to represent a new milestone or discovery.

"What was discovered during my breast cancer experience?" I pondered. Recalling our marriage vows, I realized my husband's vow to love me "in sickness and in health" had never been put to the test to the degree it had since my breast cancer diagnosis.

While my physical appearance and productivity took a nose-dive, my husband's expressions of love for me soared higher than ever. His love was likely always there, but it took the trauma of breast cancer to awaken me to its radiance. The simple yet profound truth finally sank in my diamond-hard head: My husband *loves* me.

* * *

For most of my life, I had tried to validate my existence through accomplishment. Some people would probably say I was an overachiever. I was too deceived by my misconceptions to recognize the heavy burden—the weight of trying to reach perfection—I was carrying.

I was first introduced to the idea that I was God's "beloved" three years prior to my breast cancer diagnosis. My husband and I had joined several other Christians at the home of our friends, Ted and Sylvia, for a small-group study. The book we read and discussed was *Life Of The Beloved*, by Henri J. M. Nouwen. It was extremely difficult for me to grasp the possibility that I am God's beloved child simply because *I am*. The assertion that God desired an intimate relationship with me more than He desired performance opened a door of possibility I hadn't previously considered.

While still processing and responding to this revelation, I was diagnosed with breast cancer. Sylvia suggested this daily prayer: "Lord, help me to just let you love me." She further urged me to bask in God's presence and enjoy simply allowing myself to "be" God's beloved child—a departure from my sense of needing to "do" and "serve." I found great inner peace and fulfillment in "being" with God and contemplating His love for me.

One day while recovering from a chemotherapy treatment, my eyes were drawn to a wooden bowl on our entertainment center. The bowl, created by long-time friend Dean Poe, had been crafted from a tree burl. The day I purchased the bowl at a local gift shop, I had noticed a placard placed in the display of Dean's creations that read something like this: "Imperfect bowls made by an imperfect craftsman from imperfect trees in an imperfect world." The bowls, I realized, weren't perfect, but they were distinctly beautiful and no two were alike.

As I rested on the sofa in the quiet moments of feeling weak, ill, and useless, God used the lesson brought by the wooden bowl to reveal His truth. I realized that I had mistakenly thought I had to be perfect in order to please God and others. I tried hard to be the perfect daughter, sister, friend, student, teacher, counselor, wife, mother, Christian, and now—the perfect cancer patient.

Why was I wasting my time and energy trying and failing to meet an impossible standard? A standard no one—especially God—expected of me? The chemotherapy treatment had brought with it an unexpected and amazing side effect: enlightenment to the truth that—like the bowl of wood—I am imperfect, yet distinctly beautiful, valued in my imperfection, and one of a kind. God—the Great I AM—is my Divine Craftsman, and He loves me just because "I am."

Dear Heavenly Father, I am grateful that Romans 8:28 doesn't include exemptions, such as "all things—except breast cancer—work together for good." Thank you for allowing my breast cancer to bring about good changes in me and in my relationships. I do love You and, free of my deceptions as I now am, I believe that I am Your beloved child—loved by You and others. Amen.

Regrets, Questions, and Ripple Effects

Catch the foxes for us, the little foxes that are ruining the vineyards, while our vineyards are in blossom.
—Song of Solomon 2:15

It's often the little things that seek to ruin contentment, peace of mind, and joy. While my body was recovering from the breast cancer treatments, I felt like a bud beginning to blossom—except for those "little foxes": those thoughts and happenings that were nibbling away at my long-awaited sense of well-being. Three of those little foxes in my life's vineyard were regrets, remaining questions, and ripple effects.

* * *

Regrets, regardless of whose they are or the form they take, always sadden me. Throughout my years as a prison ministry volunteer, inmates have often shared regrets. Usually their regrets include their having made choices that brought pain and grief to themselves, their families, their victims, and others. Some of the men seemed too stuck in their anger and despondency to reach beyond regret; others sought help from the community and especially from God and were able to move forward.

My having been allowed the privilege of being a confidante to several people in the retired community—as a relative, friend, or volunteer lay minister—has occasionally provided a venue to hear regrets. With misty eyes, deep sighs, and labored words, men and women have shared their heartrending regrets: a life wasted in pursuit of monetary or career success at the expense of satisfying personal relationships, taking a spouse for granted until it was too late; unwise financial decisions, destructive habits, and more. These experiences have motivated me to live my life as regret-free as possible.

That being said, my breast cancer experience has left me with the lingering regret that my husband and adult children didn't receive sufficient support. We all were thrust into new territory. None of us knew how to navigate breast cancer's course, nor even how to adequately communicate what we were feeling, thinking, and experiencing along the way.

I obtained and gave each member of my family a booklet entitled "When the Woman You Love Has Breast Cancer," but we didn't discuss the issues addressed. My husband and children seemed to handle our family crisis each in his or her own way, without the benefit of open, heart-to-heart talks about their needs and concerns.

I asked the women in a breast cancer support group for advice about this lack of openness I was pondering. An awkward silence followed. Finally, two of the women discussed how they communicated their needs to family members—but it was clear that their families had been left to flounder too.

I knew my job was to focus on my course of treatment and healing. Did my husband and children know what their job was? I doubt it. I received ample support. Their support was minimal. As a family of seemingly good communicators, we have much to learn. Our culture has much to learn.

* * *

The big unanswered question for many women diagnosed with breast cancer is "Why me?" For some reason, I never grappled with that question. A few weeks before my diagnosis, I'd been told about a woman in the community who was being treated for breast cancer. I remember thinking "It seems like every few weeks I'm hearing about another woman with breast cancer. This is getting to be like a game of Russian Roulette—you never know who's going to be next." As it turned out, I was next. I guess I didn't expect to be exempt from what was happening to so many women.

"What caused my breast cancer?" looms at the forefront of my remaining questions. I was determined to know the cause—in part so I could better comprehend my crisis, but also so I could do everything possible to prevent any responsible culprits from returning for an encore. The answer, I eventually had to concede, is elusive.

My research was as extensive as time, energy, and resources permitted. Since I am the first female in my known ancestry line to be diagnosed with breast cancer, the answer is not likely genetic predisposition. It could have been caused by inhaling, absorbing, or ingesting carcinogens from farm chemicals, a nearby landfill, cleaning supplies, and cosmetics or other personal grooming products. Perhaps foods and beverages or their containers were the cause.

Recognizing that I had overextended myself for years, resulting in an ongoing unhealthy stress level, I asked my oncologist, "Could my breast cancer have been triggered by stress?" He explained that while it is known that stress compromises immunity, and a weakened immune system has been linked to cancer, at this time it hasn't been concluded that stress causes breast cancer.

For now, the consensus seems to be the cause of breast cancer is not known. The cause could be a combination of several factors.

Now, rather than being obsessed with finding an answer that's beyond my reach, I'm concentrating on a second remaining question: "What can I do to prevent recurrence?" Finding the answer to this question has also been a challenge because there are contradictions within the information resources. While making adjustments and improvements to my diet and lifestyle, I'm encouraged by the realization that my changes are resulting in a healthier, better balanced way of life.

* * *

Ripple effects. Breast cancer is like a pebble tossed into a pool. The pebble itself seems quite small and harmless when gazed upon in one's hand. However, it is not as insignificant as it appears, because the cancer pebble is never gently dropped into the edge of the pool—it is thrown into the center with unsuspected power and causes the ripple effect of a boulder.

The first ripples of shock, fear, telling, education, and decision-making are followed by the treatment ripples. There also are a whole series of ever-widening ripples that affect meal choices and preparation, role reversals, personal plans, practical management of the treatment process, efforts to reduce and manage side effects, concerns with self-image, relationships, and daily routines, finances, careers, transportation needs, insurance, recreation, travel, and other things more difficult to identify.

You'd think the ripples caused by the breast cancer pebble would stop when the treatment ends, but no. The ripples continue to the edge of the pool—to the end of a lifetime—because the pebble has changed the composition of the pool.

As the ripples become wider and further away from the pebble, however, they can be viewed through a broader perspective. These ripples are clearer and gentler and carry new insights, priorities, dignity, resolutions, hopes, and dreams. They are actually quite beautiful and may even be looked upon as blessings.

Dear God, I yearn for the vineyard of my life to be in full blossom. I do not want regrets, questions, ripples, or anything else to ruin the bloom. Please help me quickly recognize whatever could waste away any of my days. I ask You to be the Divine Keeper of my life. Amen.

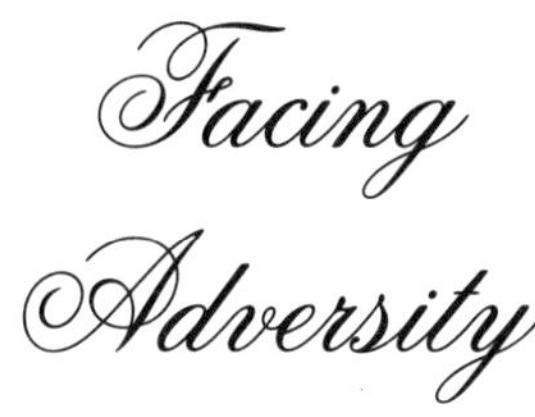

If you faint in the day of adversity,
your strength is small.
—Proverbs 24:10 (RSV)

The days progressed in a blur of jolted senses. I, along with millions of others, remained stunned during the days following September 11, 2001—the terrorist attack on our country, the United States of America. Journaling my thoughts, fears, and prayers brought me solace at that time of national crisis.

* * *

Today, I am challenged anew as I look back through my journal and read the entry written on Friday, September 14—declared to be the National Day of Prayer and Remembrance. I recall being riveted to the television, listening to the words of President George W. Bush as he spoke during the noon-hour service at the National Cathedral.

Midway through his address, some of the president's words had affected me so deeply that I had copied them into my journal from the text printed in the newspaper the next day: "It is said that adversity introduces us to ourselves. This is true of a nation as well. In this trial, we have been reminded, and the world has seen, that our fellow Americans are generous and kind, resourceful and brave."

Now, as I reread the segment of the president's speech that I'd found so profound, I personalize his words and ask myself: "Did the adversity of my breast cancer introduce me to myself?"

"Yes!" I think as I recall the scarred, hairless self I'd been forced to meet during the course of my treatment. The question, however, deserves—demands—a deeper examination and response.

Being forced to look in the face of a life-altering, potentially life-terminating foe called me to either faint in defeat or to be strong and shout the cry of victory. During the course of my battle with breast cancer, I was introduced to vulnerabilities within myself that wooed me toward surrender, but also to the emergence of an inner strength that spurred me on to conquer. "Yes," I concluded, "my breast cancer adversity did introduce me to a self that was both more vulnerable and stronger than I had previously realized."

Proverbs 24:10 proclaims, "If you faint in the day of adversity, your strength is small." With the help of God and of many people, I did not faint during my time of adversity. My spiritual, physical, and emotional strength—previously untested by a personal health crisis—grew to an extent I never would known was possible.

Quoting from a favorite childhood book, I became the "little engine that could." Picking up momentum as I chugged from, "I think I can," to, "I know I can," in overcoming my mountain of adversity, I triumphantly cheered, "I knew I could," as I began the trek down the other side.

Paging ahead in my journal, I find the next entry to be on Monday, September 17. As the New York Stock Exchange reopened that morning, President Bush's words were, "Now we all have a job to do."

What is my job for today and into my tomorrows? In part, my job is to offer into service this stronger me that I met during my breast cancer adversity. It is to do my best to nurture inner strength in my family, my friends, women experiencing breast cancer, and others—so that, with God's help, none within my sphere of influence faints in his or her day of adversity.

Dear God, I pray that Your almighty hand will guide our nation back to true allegiance to You. I pray that adversity—whether it is national or personal—would not be in vain, but would serve as a means to draw upon the increased strength that You are able to bring forth. Thank You for introducing me to my strength and enlarging it in many ways during my breast cancer affliction. Please help that strength to be "generous and kind, resourceful and brave," as I apply it in service to others. Amen.

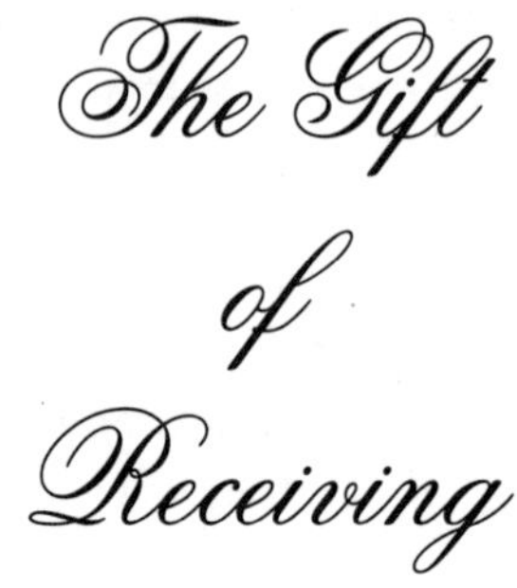

"You shall love your neighbor as yourself."

—***Matthew* 22:39**

The free gift of God is eternal life in Christ Jesus our Lord.

—***Romans* 6:23**

"It is more blessed to give than to receive" is a saying I'd heard often throughout my life. Somehow, I had drawn the erroneous conclusion that it is neither blessed nor even Christian to receive. The American culture reinforces this misconception further by placing a high value on independence that readily translates to "I should be independent and not in need of receiving from others."

My breast cancer experience prompted me to pause, swallow my pride, loose my stubborn grip on independence, and reflect on what Scripture and life experience teach about giving and receiving.

I had always tried to follow Jesus' words, "love your neighbor," by being the giver. During my months of breast cancer treatment, our "neighbors" loved their neighbors—us—as themselves. That made us the receivers.

By being on the receiving end of prayer support, medical services, encouragement, and care-giving throughout my course of treatment, I realized God was teaching me a new saying: "It is a gift to receive and to allow others the blessing of giving."

Romans 6:23 tells us the free gift of God is eternal life in Christ Jesus, our Lord. What if we are unwilling to receive this greatest gift of all? Clearly, it is God's plan for our time on earth and for eternity to be receivers as well as givers.

I have learned that gifts can sometimes come through the most unlikely channels. Breast cancer allowed me to accept the priceless gift of receiving. It is a gift I'll use and pass on to others.

Dear Heavenly Father, help me recognize and receive with grace and gratitude the love and care You give through the hands and hearts of others. Help me remember to allow others the blessing of giving. Thank You for offering Your greatest gift of all—eternal life in Christ Jesus, our Lord. I joyfully choose to honor your offer and receive Your gift. Amen.

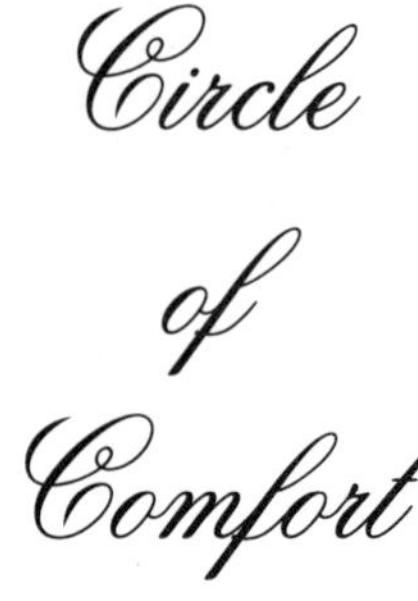

Blessed be the God and Father of our Lord Jesus Christ, the Father of mercies and God of all comfort; who comforts us in all our afflictions so that we may be able to comfort those who are in any affliction with the comfort with which we ourselves are comforted by God.

—II Corinthians 1:3-4

"Sharon! I'm so glad you're home!" my cousin Bonnie exclaimed when I responded to the ringing telephone. There was an edge of concern and urgency in her voice as we engaged in small talk. I sensed Bonnie was calling for more than chit-chat this morning.

"Sharon, one of the reasons I'm calling is because I just talked to a friend, and she told me that her family's life has been turned upside down. Her sister has been diagnosed with breast cancer. She'll be having a mastectomy tomorrow. She doesn't know anybody who has been through breast cancer treatment. I told my friend about you. Would you be willing to call her sister Judy and offer some encouragement? If so, I'll contact Judy and let her know you'll be calling," Bonnie concluded.

Of course I'll call Judy. I would have welcomed a call from a breast cancer survivor the day before my surgery—someone to offer empathy and comfort. Now that I have completed the breast cancer treatment trek, I can deeply empathize. Beyond that I am able to share comforting words, Scripture, and prayer. I can assure another person of how I experienced God's presence even during the bleakest times. I am happy to do so. It is a priority. After expressing my willingness to Bonnie, I eagerly wrote down Judy's telephone number.

As I waited, giving Bonnie time to make her introductory call to Judy, I pondered the bond—the sisterhood—among women who have experienced breast cancer. I recognized it at the breast cancer support groups I attended. I sensed it in the waiting rooms of the various treatment settings. I felt its pang when viewing a television news item or feature related to breast cancer. I was moved close to tears by it as I met other survivors while participating in a breast cancer research project. I was enriched by it through conversations and relationships with women I never would have known if we hadn't had breast cancer as our common denominator. I was overwhelmed by it when I became a part of the Komen Twin Cities Race for the Cure.

Judy would not be the first woman diagnosed with breast cancer that I'd contacted, nor would she be the last. Since my own diagnosis, there had already been three others. As I reached out to comfort as God comforts me, I experienced a great sense of joy and fulfillment in being a participant in the circle of comfort.

The circle of comfort is one of God's mysteries that I am unable to fully comprehend. There is, however, a water-pipe-and-faucet illustration that helps me better envision the afterglow of joy and fulfillment. When we as human beings participate in God's ways, we become channels of God's blessings. Just as a trace of water remains inside a water pipe and faucet after the water completes its flow, so likewise a trace of God's blessing remains in us when we allow His blessings to be channeled through us.

I've paused to pray before making my initial contact. I now am prepared to dial Judy's number. "Hello . . . ," answers a soft, tense voice. I recognize the voice. It is the voice of a sister.

Dear God and Father of our Lord Jesus Christ, You are the source of all mercy and comfort. Thank You for comforting us in our afflictions so that we may be enabled to comfort others. Thank You also for the incomprehensible joy and fulfillment You give as Your comfort is channeled through us. Thank You for the privilege of being a part of Your circle of comfort. Amen.

Transformations

And do not be conformed to this world, but be transformed by the renewing of your mind, that you may prove what the will of God is, that which is good and acceptable and perfect.

—*Romans 12:12*

Wednesday after Wednesday I'd drive by the big old yellow house on my way to the women's prayer group. Like an unsightly blemish on an otherwise attractive face, this old house on the corner was the neighborhood eyesore. The For Sale sign had been conspicuously displayed for months—maybe even a year or longer. "Who would want to invest in that forbidding monstrosity?" I'd wonder as I'd drive by. My dismay was tinged with melancholy, as I suspected the house had once been among the most respectable homes in the community.

Then one Wednesday I noticed something was changing—the For Sale sign was gone. During the next few weeks a three-story scaffold appeared on the scene and yellow paint began to disappear as it was scraped off the sides of the house. Each week the house looked uglier than the week before. As if the old peeling paint hadn't assaulted my aesthetic sense enough, now huge splotches of scraped wood flaunted their embarrassingly weathered nakedness. Age spots in the form of rusty nail-heads, moisture-erosion scars, and animal-related damage were unmasked. The old house eventually lost any remaining semblance of its bygone glory days. Every fault, flaw, and blemish was now exposed.

The next two weeks didn't seem to bring about any apparent improvement in the house. Either the workers were remaining diligent in their drudgery of repair and preparation, or they had abandoned the overwhelming project and fled in humiliation and despair.

Then one Wednesday, glancing back as I drove by, I noticed a breathtaking sight. One of the sides had been renewed. It looked fantastic. I parked my car and paused for a closer examination. The side was now painted a soft-blue hue, trimmed in off-white with burgundy accents. This house was radically changing.

Now eagerly anticipating each Wednesday morning drive-by, I was increasingly amazed as the magnificent architectural features, formerly obscured, became prominent and impressive. The transformation of this house was like a fairy tale—in fact, the house was now befitting a prince's bride.

I felt the urge to express my appreciation to those responsible for the inspiring metamorphosis but never once saw anyone at the work site. Obviously all work to date had been done other times than Wednesday mornings.

* * *

Today as I drove by, I observed playground equipment and outdoor toys. Then my glance was drawn to movement next to the house. Someone was putting the finishing touches on the final side. I had to stop and express my thoughts to whoever had the vision, skills, and perseverance to restore this house.

Noticing me, a young woman left her perch beside the house and approached. "I just wanted to tell you what a blessing it has been to watch the transformation of this house," I explained. "Why, thank you!" the woman beamed as she gave me a spontaneous hug. Hugging her back I said, "You saw beyond the flaws in this house and imagined its potential. You've made it one of the most beautiful homes in the community. God bless you!" "God bless you too," she replied as she told me about the vision she and her husband had for the house.

Brimming over with lingering joy as I drove away, I contemplated my encounter with the woman and the house she and her husband had transformed. My thoughts meandered to my breast cancer experience. Like that house, I also had faults, flaws, and blemishes hidden below the surface. My breast cancer experience was serving as a means to scrape away the outer façade and expose my vulnerabilities.

Some would have perceived me as hopelessly unattractive—an eyesore not worth an investment. But God, like the young couple with the house, is a visionary. He is the Divine Visionary Who knew that even something like breast cancer could be used in positive ways to transform me by the renewing of not only my mind, but also my body, emotions, spirit, and relationships.

I am now a breast cancer survivor. In what ways has breast cancer changed me? Within the ongoing transformation process, I believe I am becoming less conformed to this temporal world. Rather than succumbing to societal pressures and expectations, I am more discriminating. I am asking myself questions such as these: Is this opinion or practice consistent with Scripture? Will it enhance or hinder the relationships that are most important to me? What is the motivating factor? If it is social acceptance or prestige, what is the price? Is it worth the price?

Part of my renewal is a conscious longing to live my life according to the will of God. I am committed to intentionally seeking and confirming God's will through praying, studying of Scripture, seeking the counsel of mature Christians, reading related books by Christian authors, and by other means I learn of. After all, it was God who invested in me through the giving of His Son, Jesus. He paid the ultimate price so that renewal and change could be possible for me and for others who will accept His ultimate gift.

Dear God, I believe that Your will for me is that which is good and acceptable and perfect. Help me not to be conformed to this world in ways that fall short of Your will. I ask that You continue to transform me by renewing my mind so that I am able to discern Your will. Thank You for investing in me. Amen.

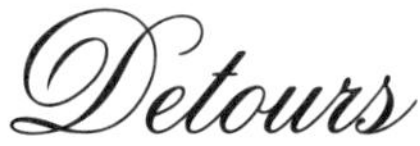

Be strong and courageous! Do not tremble or be dismayed, for the Lord your God is with you wherever you go.
—Joshua 1:9

The framed photograph of my father again captures my attention as I walk through our family room. I cherish this recently received picture of my now-deceased dad. I recall struggling to hold back tears the day I first spotted it—one among many old pictures in my cousin Bonnie's collection of family photographs. Sensing my longing for the photo, Bonnie generously made a copy for herself and sent me the original.

My dad, so striking and handsome at the age of twenty-two—no wonder he seized my mother's heart. Today, though, I am looking beyond the features of the young man who became my father. I am contemplating the expression in his face, particularly his eyes. He looks so peaceful, so content, so optimistic. I wonder what his young-man hopes and dreams were as he posed for this photograph on that long-ago day.

My mother said she had seen the photograph before. She recognized it as a passport photo taken when Dad applied for a government overseas construction project. There never was a passport, however, and Dad never was able to follow through with his intended plan. Instead, his life journey took an unplanned detour. Pearl Harbor was attacked, the United States of America was swept into World War II, and Dad was drafted into the army.

The small-town Minnesota farm boy, training to be a soldier at a base in faraway New York, persuaded his hometown sweetheart to take the long bus trip east to join him in marriage. I was conceived a few months later, just before he was shipped overseas. Farm boy, draftee, husband, father-to-be, soldier. The young man's detour took him to North Africa and Italy—to a battleground of endurance, a struggle for survival, and a longing to return to life as before.

Shortly after I celebrated my second birthday, my soldier-daddy came back to Minnesota—home to Mom and me. He came home a changed man. There could be no true returning to life as before. Though still a young man in his twenties, Dad had acquired emotional scars during his detour. He also had gleaned wisdom beyond his years—wisdom that he passed on to me and to others.

I, too, have experienced an unplanned, life-changing detour. My breast cancer detour has also been a battle to endure, a struggle to survive, and a longing to return to life as before. I, too, have been changed by my unexpected detour. I, too, am left with scars. I, too, have gleaned wisdom beyond my years. It took my own detour to allow me to understand and appreciate the wisdom Dad passed on to his family after his detour—that life and freedom are precious and fragile and should never be taken for granted. He believed in being cautious before making commitments that carry unhealthy stress, in cherishing people and the simple pleasures in life, and in enjoying and nurturing God's creation.

A detour is a deviation from one's usual route, often a path taken around some obstacle or danger. Along my own detour, I have encountered obstacles and dangers. I don't want my ordeal to have been in vain.

Like Dad and like the countless multitudes before me whose life journeys have taken detours, I have become a wiser person. It behooves me to share what I have gained—through the telling of the self-examination, insights, and positive changes brought forth through my experience, and through a life better lived.

Dear God, I would prefer my life to be predictable, safe, and within my control. If left to my choosing, I would not have ventured on a life-changing detour. However, detours are not always left to choice. Thank You for not leaving me to stumble alone along my detour, trembling and dismayed. Thank You for promising to be with me wherever I go. With You, I am able to be strong and courageous in the face of the obstacles and dangers I encounter. Through You, I am able to know that detours need not be in vain. Please show me how best to apply in my own life, and how best to share with others, the wisdom I have gained. Amen.

Carried by Prayer

Evening, and morning, and at noon, will I pray, and cry aloud: and He shall hear my voice.

—Psalm 55:17 (KJV)

Devote yourselves to prayer, keeping alert in it with an attitude of thanksgiving.

—Colossians 4:22

Be joyful in hope, patient in affliction, faithful in prayer.

—Romans 12:12

I've known about prayer for as long as I can remember. Over the years, I've come to believe in prayer and I've done a lot of praying. But just when I think I've learned all there is to know about it, I find myself learning something fresh, significant, and powerful.

My breast cancer diagnosis ushered in an unprecedented awareness that I was becoming the recipient of many prayers from many people that would continue for a long time. From my diagnosis day on, I knew I was being prayed for. Whether stated directly or promised in a greeting card, the words "I'm praying for you," always encouraged and blessed me. Although I felt I was "carried by prayer" throughout my breast cancer experience, certain prayers and certain settings were especially significant and powerful. Some are revisited in the devotional "Healing," and others are shared as follows:

Shortly after my first surgery, my husband, my children, and I attended a family reunion. Cousins from several states and from Europe joined my Minnesota relatives for a large gathering of our family clan. My cousin Dean was undergoing treatment for esophagus cancer and was unable to attend. After the picnic dinner, Dean's wife, Betty, welcomed my pastor brother-in-law, Keith, a few other relatives, and me into their home to visit Dean. When Keith offered to lead a prayer for our healing, Dean and I sat side by side, with family members gathered around us. The prayers that followed transcended kinship—Dean and I were God's beloved children, willing recipients of His healing.

* * *

"Val is in town, so I'm having a few women from church here for the afternoon." Diane sounded excited as she invited me to join the gathering. My enthusiasm matched hers because I relished the opportunity to spend time with Val, a former member of the congregation who had moved out of state. The problem was, I had a postoperative appointment with my surgeon the same afternoon. After I'd explained my dilemma to Diane, we decided I would attend the get-together for as long as possible before leaving for my appointment.

As I had anticipated, the afternoon was a delightful time of reminiscing and catching up on each other's lives. As my time to depart neared, one of the women asked me to give the group an update on my treatment status. I welcomed the opportunity to do so. I also mentioned my anxiety about the appointment that would transpire in less than an hour. I explained that because Colin and I had decided on a less extensive second surgery procedure than the one that the surgeon had recommended, I was worried that our decision would compromise the positive rapport we had previously established with him.

As the women and I formed a circle of clasped hands, Diane brought our united desire for God's guidance to Him in prayer. I took my leave knowing that the prayers of my sisters in the church family had reached our Heavenly Father. The prayer was answered beyond my highest hopes, as recounted in the "Second Opinion—Second Surgery" devotional.

⁂

It was shortly before Christmas, and I had recently completed the fourth of eight chemotherapy treatments. Although I was grateful to be carried through my treatments by the prayers of others, I was sensing a vague lack of fulfillment in my own prayer life. Feeling nauseated, fatigued, and discouraged, I decided to accompany my husband on a shopping trip to a Christian bookstore in the hope that the brief outing would lift my sagging spirit.

As I stood next to my husband in the checkout line, I noticed a framed print displayed on a nearby wall. Drawn to it, I stepped out of line and walked over to view the print more closely. The woman depicted in the print was the epitome of feminine loveliness as she knelt in prayer before an open Bible. She embodied the beauty, grace, and devotion I was feeling totally devoid of. I could no longer hold back my brimming emotions and began to quietly weep.

Noticing my tears, a woman left her place in line, walked over to me and gently said, "You're supposed to have that print. Please accept my store coupon. Perhaps it will help you be able to purchase it." Choking back my tears and surprise, I thanked her. My husband used the coupon to purchase the print as part of my Christmas gift. God had heard my unspoken yearning, and initiated His answer through the generosity of the woman and my husband.

I learned that the print, entitled "He Shall Hear My Voice," had been painted by C. Michael Dudash. In referring to his painting, Dudash has written, "I have attempted to convey a particular sense of timelessness and a place 'in the spirit' with this painting—we're not sure if it's morning, noon, or early evening . . . if she's in a sunlit room or a porch in the open air . . . if she is happy or sad, if she's giving thanks or beseeching the Lord for some great need. . . . As you meditate on this print, I pray you will be motivated to seek the Lord and find through your own prayer life, a place of rest in Him."

I now believe the reason God blesses me through the print isn't the woman's feminine beauty, as I had first thought. Rather, I believe it to be the deep, fulfilling, prayer life she portrays. My breast cancer experience has brought me to a personal prayer life that is an ongoing dialogue with God—like, and yet beyond, what I am able to experience with an intimate companion. The conversation may be spoken, in my thoughts, or sung. It may be silent contemplation, a basking in God's presence, or journal writing. It is unrehearsed and spontaneous. My words may not be eloquent, but they express what I truly want to say. My expressions of emotion may not always be pleasing to God, but I know He receives them because they are what I am genuinely feeling.

* * *

I've come to realize that my longing to be loved for myself—rather than for what I can do or give—is a reflection of God's heart. I believe God is pleased when I seek to just be with Him—to enjoy His company as He enjoys mine. I understand more fully what it means to be carried by prayer.

Dear Father God, the realization that You are eager to hear the voice of Your children evening, morning, at noon, and any time, calls me to devotion and thanksgiving. Thank You for those whose prayers helped carry me through my season of breast cancer. Because of Who You are, I can continue to be joyful in hope, patient in affliction, and faithful in prayer. Amen.

Healing

Is anyone among you sick? Let him call for the elders of the church, and let them pray over him, anointing him with oil in the name of the Lord; and the prayer offered in faith will restore the one who is sick.

—James 5:14,15

He Himself bore our sins in His body on the cross, that we might die to sin and live to righteousness: for by His wounds you were healed.

—1 Peter 2:24

It wasn't until I became desperate for my own healing that I thought much about whether or not God still heals as He did in Biblical times. That happened when I was a new mother breast-feeding my infant. I was plagued by recurring acute-bacterial-infection-caused mastitis—mastitis being an inflammation of tissue in the breast.

My sister Carol suggested I attend a healing service at a church she had heard about in Minneapolis. During the days prior to the upcoming Wednesday service, I read every New Testament reference to healing, and my faith grew in the process.

I attended the service as I'd planned and heeded the pastor's invitation to come to the altar for prayer. When he touched my head and prayed, I saw a brilliant white light within my closed eyelids. A tingling sensation moved from my toes to my chest, and culminated with a sense that I was breathing in fresh, healing air and breathing out the mastitis. I knew God had healed me, and so it proved to be—the disease never returned.

Carol and my husband and a few others rejoiced with me and praised God for the healing. When I perceived some people to be uncomfortable with my healing testimony, however, I discontinued telling others about the experience, and I thought about it less and less as the years went by.

Almost thirty years later, I was meeting with a small group of friends to plan a Christian-growth retreat. When I told the group members of my breast cancer diagnosis and upcoming surgery, they gathered around me, laid hands on me, and prayed. I gladly received not only their prayers, but also a simultaneous insight from God.

God was reminding me that both serious illnesses during my life have involved my breasts. While my friends prayed for me, I sensed that—although God could heal my breast through Divine intervention as before—this time it was His plan to use medical personnel and procedures. I was filled with an inner assurance that I was proceeding according to God's will for me.

Shortly after my surgery, I learned that a local church, was hosting a national conference and would be having guest pastors speak at the evening services. The services were open to the public, and one evening I followed my strong desire to attend. One of the pastors followed his message with the invitation to the listeners to come forward for individual prayer. Hesitantly, I walked forward, unsure of how I should phrase my prayer request.

I didn't need to voice my request, however, because he seemed to already have the knowledge he needed. He spoke to the congregation, saying, "This woman needs prayer for an infirmity in her body." Those present joined the pastor in praying that God would heal my infirmity.

Several days later, I discussed the healing prayer—and the knowledge it seemed God had given the pastor—with several women in my weekly prayer group. We came to an understanding that God knew there were cancer cells remaining somewhere in my body following the breast surgery and we believed those remaining cells—the infirmity—had been destroyed by prayer.

"What about my planned course of treatment—a second surgery, chemotherapy, and radiation treatment?" I wondered aloud. Should I accept that I had been totally healed and refuse the prescribed course of treatment? As the women and I prayed, we were unified in our belief that I was to proceed with the planned treatments—that the course of treatment would serve a purpose.

Only later did I realize that God would call me to write a devotional book for women experiencing breast cancer. I now believe it was important for me to personally walk the treatment path that many women with breast cancer must experience. I have begun to understand that our sovereign God, in His infinite love and wisdom, at times has a purpose higher than Divine healing. Recently my friend Eileen relayed to me this very appropriate quote from an unknown source: God permits in His wisdom what He could prevent in His power.

Dreams had rarely held much interest for me—until one that I had shortly after completing the course of my treatment for breast cancer. When I awoke from the dream, I knew it had come from God, and that it carried significance and purpose.

In the dream, I was observing birds in the trees and the sky. They were beautiful, healthy birds—living life to the fullest. They were content, making their cheery bird sounds as they found food, built nests, socialized, and cared for their young. Watching them filled me with joy.

Then I glanced at the ground. It, too, was full of birds—even more than I'd seen in trees and sky. Examining the birds on the ground, I realized they all had broken wings of varying severity. Like the ones in the trees and sky, these birds, too, were finding food, building nests, socializing, and caring for their young. They were doing their best to fully their lives while being confined to the ground.

Contemplating the dream, I asked God to help me understand its meaning and purpose. The insight came to me that the birds were to be likened to people—His children of all ages—who were emotionally and spiritually wounded. God then brought to my remembrance the Raptor Center in Minnesota. I knew the Raptor Center to be a place where wounded birds of prey, such as eagles, are brought for human-assisted healing, and are then returned to their natural habitat. God gave me the realization that just as He can use people in the healing of birds, He also can use people in the healing of His children.

Later, I asked God another question through prayer, "Why were some birds whole and healthy while others were wounded?" The thought that came to my mind startled me. It was this: *All* of the birds I saw in the dream had been wounded at some point—the birds that were able to soar and live life to the fullest were healed birds.

So often I, along with many others, equate healing with a physical condition. God made it clear to me that emotional and spiritual healing are also necessary for individual wholeness.

Reviewing my life, I realize that God has been in the process of healing my own emotional and spiritual wounds. He has used many means and people in my ongoing healing. I am aware that as I am healed in certain areas, God enables me to be one of His channels of healing for people with similar wounds.

Whether physically, emotionally, or spiritually wounded, we are being healed—not only for our own benefit, but also for the benefit of others.

Dear Sovereign God, I'm grateful You are the Divine Healer. Help me trust in You and Your higher purpose for whatever form Your healing of me and others may take. Please help me remain teachable and receptive, so that I am able to experience healing and be used as a channel for Your healing of others. Thank You for the wounds Jesus bore on the cross for my sins, so that through my belief in Him, I can be healed for eternity. Amen.

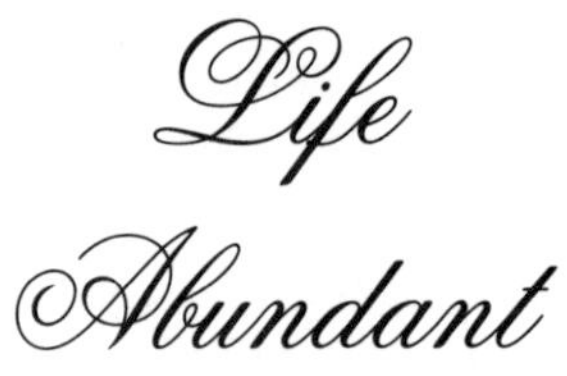

Life Abundant

I came that they might have life, and might have it abundantly.

—John 10:10

I was beginning to take life for granted again. It had been twenty-six months since my breast cancer diagnosis. I was over three months into my second year as a breast cancer survivor. Life finally felt normal again and I was becoming complacent in my vow to cherish and revere each and every day of life.

But then, as the summer wound down, the veterinarian informed us that our dog Mandy's life was waning. She was over twelve and a half years old—a ripe old age for a German shepherd. My husband and I had been in denial, refusing to accept the reality that Mandy's life was nearing its end. During the summer we had spent enough on veterinary bills to replace her with a new registered purebred German shepherd. There could, however, be no new purebred German shepherd registered under the name of our Mandolin Dandy.

The time had come to deal with the truth. Mandy would likely not recover from her ailments. Her fur had lost its luster—and it could no longer conceal her alarming weight loss. It was obviously a struggle for her to maneuver her weak, arthritic body from resting place to resting place. We would need the services of the veterinarian and his assistant one more time. The telephone call was made. The appointment was set. Dr. Pedersen and an assistant would be at our farm at 11:00 Saturday morning. The beat-by-beat of Mandy's life-sustaining heart would now be measured by the second-by-second tick of a clock.

* * *

Today is the Saturday. I have a million and one things to do, but the one is more important than the million. My priority until 11:00 is to be with Mandy—to lavish her with love and appreciation. Too weak to accompany me as usual to her spot near my lawn chair, Mandy instead welcomes my joining her near the house where she is resting. She is refusing food and water today, but seems content as I stroke her fur and sooth her with loving words.

As I stroke her, Mandy's life plays in my mind like a movie nearing its final scene. Our son Aaron picked her out of a litter during his first year at college. Within weeks she won the hearts of our family and over the years expanded her loving sphere to include almost everyone who came to our farm. It amazes me to realize that, aside from an occasional trip to the vet or some other brief outing, Mandy has lived her whole life on this farm that she claimed while a pup. Seasons came and went as she participated in the activities of those entering her domain. When home alone, Mandy lay on the front porch and assumed her duty as watchdog. As dogs go, Mandy has lived an abundant life.

Hearing a vehicle enter our driveway, I check my watch. With a sigh of relief, I see the time is only 10:00—the vehicle won't be the veterinarian's. It is my son-in-law, Vince, and his son—my grandson—Hudson.

Hudson, almost two, wants to feed Mandy and brings a handful, then two more, of food from her bowl. To our surprise, Mandy stands and eats Hudson's offering—both are oblivious to the meaning within this simple act. In a sense, this last meal is symbolic of the cycle of life. Twelve years ago Mandy was the frisky youngster pup exploring the wonders of this farm. Today she receives her final nourishment from the hand of this exuberant young child who now takes his turn discovering Mandy's former kingdom.

Soon after Vince and Hudson leave, my husband, Colin, returns from his morning meeting and joins me at Mandy's side. It is 10:30 now. My tears flow freely as I savor life—Mandy's life. I feel the warmth of her aliveness and take pleasure in her gaze of affection, the slight movements and sounds she makes. She knows she is loved. I wonder if she senses that life, for her, is almost over.

Another vehicle is now approaching. Yes, it is time, and Dr. Pedersen and Caroline drive in. Aware of the significance of their task, their demeanor is respectful and compassionate. The four of us walk across the farmyard with Mandy slowly following behind. Colin leads the way to the burial site he prepared early this morning. I thank God for the beautiful day and find comfort in the radiant sunlight filtering through the canopy of leaves.

Mandy dutifully lies down beside her final bed. The veterinarian and his assistant kneel beside her. Within seconds, Mandy's eyes close and Dr. Pedersen confirms that her heart has ceased beating. He and his assistant leave, considerate in allowing Colin and me privacy to embrace before dealing with Mandy's lifeless body, our grief, our memories, and eventually our last words. "Thank you, Mandy, for sharing your life, your unconditional love, your one-of-a-kind personality, your loyalty, your service, your final lesson." Life, whether a pet's or a human being's, is precious and fragile. Life is to be lived today—because eventually there will not be another day to live. Life is to be lived abundantly.

> **Dear God, You are the creator and giver of life. Through Your Divine provision, Jesus Christ came that I may have life and have it abundantly. Please forgive me when I take Your gift of life for granted. May my desires and actions each day be in accordance with the prayer Jesus taught, "Thy will be done on earth as it is in heaven," so that I don't settle for less than the abundant life that is available through You. Amen.**

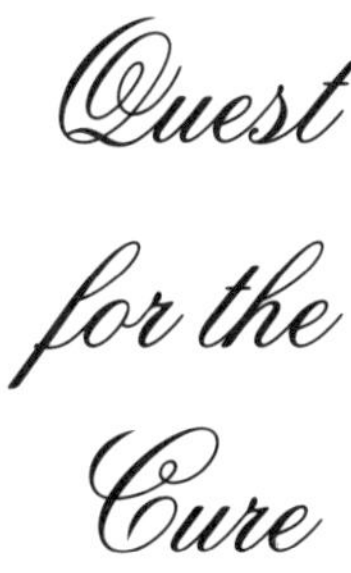

Let us therefore draw near with confidence to the throne of grace, that we may receive mercy and find grace to help in time of need.

—Hebrews 4:16

A calendar in the mailbox captures my attention at once. Whether intentionally or not, the cover provides a portrait that is of inspiration to women experiencing breast cancer—those currently undergoing treatment, those who are survivors, and the multitudes who worry about a possible future diagnosis.

The cover photograph places the viewer in the center of a straight, tree-lined country lane that continues into the distance for as far as the eye can see. The lushness of the grass bordering the path and the freshness of the leaves' green hue suggest that the picture was taken during the springtime.

Although the trees at first glance appear perfect in their beauty, a closer look reveals scars where branches have been removed. Twigs and small branches on the ground provide proof that the trees have withstood the winds of storms. One of the trees in the forefront bears an injury at the base of its trunk, as well as evidence of a disruption to the earth that anchors its hidden source of strength and nourishment—its roots.

The sun's brilliance is carried beyond the picturesque setting, and warms not only the dappled pathway but the soul of the onlooker as well. In the distance, a bright-green strip divides the narrow gravel road lengthwise—testifying to the grass seeds' victorious persistence in pressing toward life-giving sun and rain.

Now, as I contemplate the setting, I understand its power to captivate me. I see—not trees—but a line of women marching into the distance that is beyond my view. The trees in the forefront I liken to recently diagnosed women, just beginning their journey down Breast Cancer Lane. Along the path are those women who are progressing further and further into their course of treatment.

Just as the tree-lined path extends beyond the onlooker's limited view, so does the regiment of women continue farther and farther into the distance. These women are the survivors of breast cancer. Some of the women have forgotten how far they have traveled, and they pause to count their years of survival before continuing on their way.

These women in the distance offer great inspiration and encouragement to those following behind—for they have been victorious over the storms that disfigured and scarred, and the elements that poisoned, burned, and attempted to destroy their life-sustaining roots. If I strain my ears, perhaps I'll hear them calling back, "Carpe diem! Yes, seize the day—for each day lived fully while you are on Breast Cancer Lane carries with it the possibility of weeks, months, and years of fulfillment ahead."

I am ready to draw my attention away from the photograph, when I realize that there is more to this setting than meets the eye. A pressing question comes to my mind: "What is lining the lane *behind* my view?" Could it be the seeds of trees that sooner or later will join those already there? If so, those trees, as yet unseen, represent the hundreds of thousands of women who will be diagnosed with breast cancer in the years to come—unless a cure is found.

A pang of urgency grips me as I long to spare others from having to take a place on the path. It is true that Breast Cancer Lane does have a beauty of its own and that there are valuable lessons to be gained by a journey down its path. Nevertheless, such beauty and valuable lessons could be found in other settings. I want a cure to be found, and a barrier to be placed across the lane. I want to help hang a huge sign that proclaims *Entrance Permanently Blocked.*

Feeling small and insignificant alongside such a huge challenge, I sigh and ask myself, "What can one woman do in the quest for a breast cancer cure?" Then I remember a story I read in my e-mail months ago, "The Daffodil Principle." The woman telling the story relates the events that unfolded when she accompanies her daughter, Carolyn, on an outing. She writes

* * *

> *After about twenty minutes, we turned onto a small gravel road and saw a hand-lettered sign that read, 'Daffodil Garden.' . . . As we turned a corner of the path I looked up and gasped. Before me lay the most glorious sight. It looked as though someone had taken a great vat of gold and poured it down over the mountain peak and slopes . . . There were five acres of flowers.*
>
> *"But who has done this?" I asked Carolyn. "It's just one woman," Carolyn answered. "That's her home." On the patio, we saw a poster. "Answers to the Questions I know You Are Asking" was the headline. The first answer was a simple one: 50,000 bulbs, it read. The second answer was: One at a time, by one woman.*

The leaflet concluded with the question, "What has God laid on your heart?" I pondered the principle so beautifully brought to my awareness through the daffodil story: If each person does even one act at a time, the sum of all of the acts can be amazing.

Applying the daffodil principle and the question posed in the leaflet, I asked myself, "What has God laid on my heart related to the challenge of conquering breast cancer?"

- I could encourage and support women currently experiencing breast cancer.
- I could participate in clinical or research studies.
- I could assist financially in the promotion of education, support systems, political lobbying, or research through direct giving or fundraisers.

As Christians, we must not overlook the power of prayer. As God's children, we are invited to "draw near with confidence to His throne of grace" to find help "in time of need." Let's be a multitude seeking help from the One Who can lead us to the cure. Let it not be said of us, of me, as it is in James 4:20, "You do not have because you do not ask."

> **Dear Father, I believe You are the One all-knowing, always-present, omnipotent, merciful, and loving God. I come with confidence to Your throne of grace, asking You to help find the cure for breast cancer. I thank You for hearing my prayer, and I wait with trusting expectancy for Your answer. To You be the praise and glory. Amen.**

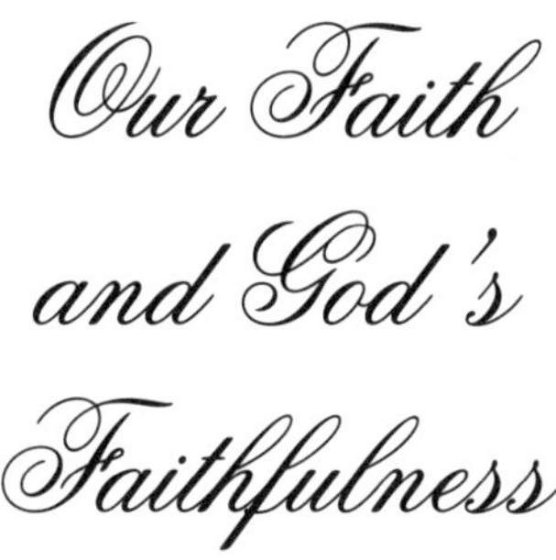

If we are faithless, He remains faithful; for He cannot deny Himself.
—II Timothy 2:13

The Lord's loving kindnesses indeed never cease, for His compassions never fail. They are new every morning; Great is Thy Faithfulness.
—Lamentations 3:22,23

"Picture of Innocence" would be an appropriate title for the photograph on our living room wall. The framed scene has captured a moment in time during a winter day long ago. Three children are walking hand in hand through a wooded winter wonderland; the red-mittened toddler in the middle clutching the hands of the older children at his sides. Walking away from the viewer, the bundled children trudge through the woods toward a bend in the path—oblivious to their trail of boot-prints in the virgin snow.

Waves of nostalgia sweep over me as I gaze misty-eyed at the children in the photograph—our children. Toddler Matthew's faith is in his sister, Krissy, and his brother, Aaron, as the three venture into unexplored territory within their grandpa's woods.

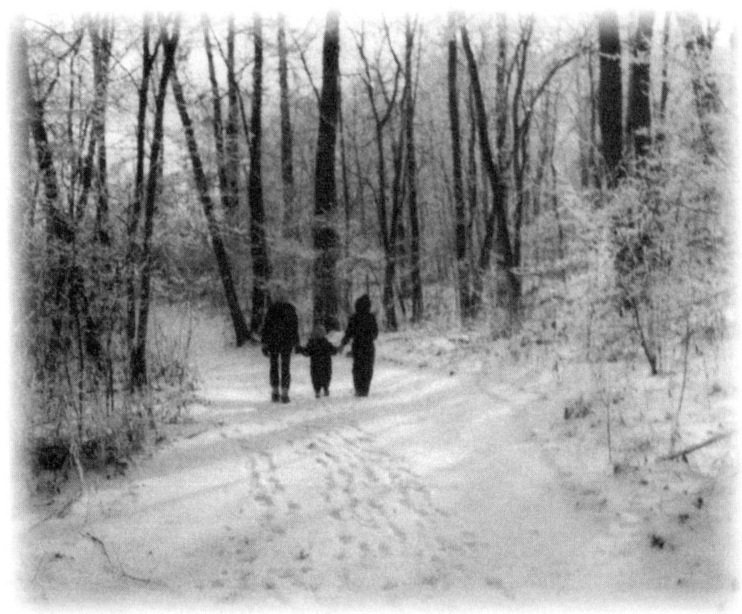

Our children are all adults now. They—as did my husband and I before them—have lost their childlike innocence while navigating through a world that is often unpredictable, challenging, painful, and potentially destructive. What do we have to offer our children? What can we teach them so that they will not only survive, but also thrive while living in this world? The answer to these questions for me, reached in part through my breast cancer experience, is twofold: faith and God's faithfulness.

As we are assured in II Timothy, God's faithfulness is not dependent on our faith. Although I still have a long way to go, my own faith in God has gradually matured as my history of personally experiencing His faithfulness has expanded. I would like to share with others how my experience with breast cancer strengthened my faith and revealed new dimensions of God's faithfulness.

Loss of innocence comes in part with the realization that bad things can and do happen. Faith in God does not bring an exemption from bad things. I have come to believe, however, that I can place my faith in God because, as promised in Romans 8:28, He is faithful in causing all things—even bad things—"to work for good to those who love God, to those who are called according to His purpose."

Not only is God able to bring good out of bad, He also is faithful to His promise in Hebrews 11:1, "Never will I leave you, never will I forsake you." I have found that at times I clearly sense God's presence with me. But I can be assured through faith in His word that He is *always* with me, whether or not I feel His presence. Even those who love us most let us down or desert us at times, but God is always faithful.

Our greatest challenge can be in our own minds—the anxious, fearful, worst-case-scenario thoughts that enter and persist. If unchecked, such thoughts can become a crippling obsession. God displays His faithfulness by providing guidance through Scripture. I found an answer to my own tormenting mind games in 2 Corinthians 10:3-5, especially in the phrase, "taking every thought captive to the obedience of Christ."

When I catch myself thinking debilitating thoughts, I pause to consider their source. If the thoughts aren't consistent with Scripture or God's character as revealed through Scripture, I realize the thoughts are coming from my own human imagination or possibly even from Satan. I prayerfully give the disturbing thoughts to God, asking Him to relieve me of them—to take them captive. Next, I read faith-nurturing Scripture verses, such as II Timothy 1:7 (KJV): "For God has not given us the spirit of fear; but of power, and of love, and of a sound mind."

My breast cancer experience has brought me closer than I once was to the state of contentment described by the Apostle Paul in Philippians 4:11-13. My growing faith is enabling me to declare, like Paul, "I can do all things through Him who strengthens me."

One of the most unexpected benefits that came through my breast cancer journey is that of overcoming my fear of death. I came to grips with my mortality when the CT scan, a procedure done prior to my first radiation treatment, revealed a spot on my liver. Since the ultrasound appointment that would determine the nature of the spot was a week away, I had seven days to deal with the possibility that I could have liver cancer.

When I could no longer overcome my fearful thoughts by reading Scripture or any other means, I went before God in prayer and gave Him my body. I imagined myself willingly climbing on an altar and relinquishing myself to God. A deep inner peace and yearning to be with God in heaven followed my prayer.

As it turned out, the ultrasound procedure performed later identified the spot as a small, harmless cyst.

The scare I encountered that week is now only a memory, but the anticipation of someday being with God in heaven remains and has overtaken my fear of death. I am able to personalize the words found in Ecclesiastes 5:20, "For I will not often consider the years of my life, because God keeps me occupied with the gladness of my heart."

"Great Is Thy Faithfulness," by Thomas Chisholm and William Runyan, has become one of my favorite hymns. Based on the words found in the third chapter of Lamentations, the hymn assures us of God's faithfulness during all seasons—summer and winter, springtime and harvest. God is faithful throughout all the seasons we experience during life—the inevitable changes, the mountaintop times, and the valleys of struggle, pain, and crisis.

As I write this final devotional of praise to God for His faithfulness during my breast cancer season, my family is entering a new season of challenge. The innocent toddler depicted in "Picture of Innocence" is now a twenty-five-year-old U.S. Army reservist recently deployed to hazardous duty service, leaving a training base in his homeland for an undisclosed, classified mission in an undisclosed, classified faraway destination. Grandson Hudson is the toddler in our family now—innocent and unaware of life's perils as he gleefully plants slobbery farewell kisses on his Uncle Matt's face.

This devotional is not just my story or our family story—it is everyone's story.

Sooner or later, generation after generation, all of us lose our innocent faith in a wonderland world. We need to know whose hand to hold and in whom to place our faith. As God's children, we are invited to hold our Father's hand, and to place our faith in His loving-kindnesses that never cease and compassions that never fail.

Dear Faithful God, You created the seasons of nature and the seasons of life—neither being free of storms. As a new season unfolds and a new day dawns, I join generations before me in singing the chorus, "Great is Thy faithfulness! Great is Thy faithfulness! Morning by morning new mercies I see. All I have needed Thy hand hath provided. Great is Thy faithfulness, Lord unto me." Amen.

Afterword

As *On Wings of the Dawn* goes to the printer, I am celebrating being a two-year breast cancer survivor. One of the most amazing and fulfilling outcomes of my breast cancer experience continues to be the opportunity to support others—especially women experiencing breast cancer or some other crisis.

More and more, the wings of the dawn are carrying me to places where I am privileged to offer encouragement and hope to both women and men. It may be over the telephone, through a greeting card or e-mail, or in a one-on-one visit or a speaking engagement.

While the writing of this book is coming to a close, I sense God is calling me to further ministry with women and those who support them. Already, I believe God is nudging me with topics to be addressed. An excitement and passion is mounting within me as I ponder the topics being conceived in my mind, heart, and soul that will—in God's time and way—be developed for the purpose of bringing support and hope to others in a variety of settings.

I am more convinced than ever that breast cancer—or any kind of crisis experience—is not to be grieved as a wasted season in life. Rather, a crisis holds the possibility of the survivor someday being able to call back with deep empathy and compassion to those in a similar situation.

My last message to you is expressed through these words from the classic devotional book, *Streams in the Desert*, by Mrs. Charles E. Cowman. First printed in 1925, they capture the timelessness of the "calling back" mission offered to you and to me:

Life is a steep climb, and it does the heart good to have somebody "call back" and cheerily beckon us on up the high hill. We are all climbers together, and we must help one another. This mountain climbing is serious business, but glorious. It takes strength and steady step to find the summits. The outlook widens with the altitude. If anyone among us has found anything worthwhile, we ought to "call back."

If you have gone a little way ahead of me, call back—'Twill cheer my heart and help my feet along the stony track; And if, perchance, Faith's light is dim, because the oil is low, Your call will guide my lagging course as wearily I go.

Call back, and tell me that He went with you into the storm; Call back, and say He kept you when the forest's roots were torn; That, when the heaven's thunder and the earthquake shook the hill, He bore you up and held you where the very air was still.

Oh, friend, call back, and tell me for I cannot see your face; They say it glows with triumph, and your feet bound in the race; But there are mists between us and my spirit eyes are dim, And I cannot see the glory, though I long for word of Him.

But if you'll say He heard you, when your prayer was but a cry, And if you'll say He saw you through the night's sin-darkened sky—If you have gone a little way ahead, oh friend, call back—'Twill cheer my heart and help my feet along the stony track.

About the Author

Sharon Callister was diagnosed with breast cancer in 2000. Her life experiences include high school counseling, teaching, and serving as a missionary at an international school in Japan. She was the founding director of Shepherd's Center of the Cannon Valley, an interdenominational service organization for senior adults. Committed to volunteerism, she is especially dedicated to prison ministry, mentoring, and more recently, supporting women and men encountering cancer.

Sharon Callister and her husband, Colin, have four grown children. Except for the past five school terms spent living in the suburb of Woodbury, they have made their home in rural Cannon falls, Minnesota. An experienced public speaker, she welcomes requests for speaking engagements, as well as comments from readers, at *whispering_hope_ministries@earthlink.net*.

Subjects Index

Order Form

To purchase additional copies of *On Wings of the Dawn*, please fill out the form below:

Number of Books:	________	x	$16.95	_________
Shipping/Handling	per book	x	2.95	_________
Sales Tax (MN residents only)	per book	x	.97	_________
			Total	_________

Ship to:

Name:____

Address:____

City:_______________ State:______________ Zip:_________

Phone: ____

Make Checks payable to: ***Whispering Hope Ministries***

If you would like Sharon to insert a personalized message, please include that here:

____

____

____

Mail or fax your order to:

Sharon Callister
27148 Inga Ave.
Cannon Falls, MN 55009

Fax: 507-263-2218